Breastfeeding and
the Pursuit of Happiness

Breastfeeding and the Pursuit of Happiness

PHYLLIS L.F. RIPPEY

McGill-Queen's University Press

Montreal & Kingston | London | Chicago

ISBN 978-0-2280-0885-9 (cloth)
ISBN 978-0-2280-1015-9 (ePDF)

Legal deposit fourth quarter 2021
Bibliothèque nationale du Québec

Printed in Canada on acid-free paper that is 100% ancient forest free
(100% post-consumer recycled), processed chlorine free

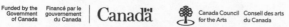

We acknowledge the support of the Canada Council for the Arts.

Nous remercions le Conseil des arts du Canada de son soutien.

Library and Archives Canada Cataloguing in Publication

Title: Breastfeeding and the pursuit of happiness / Phyllis L.F.
    Rippey.
Names: Rippey, Phyllis L. F., author.
Description: Includes bibliographical references and index.
Identifiers: Canadiana (print) 20210248718 | Canadiana
    (ebook) 20210248777 | ISBN 9780228008859 (hardcover) |
    ISBN 9780228010159 (PDF)
Subjects: LCSH: Breastfeeding. | LCSH: Breastfeeding—Social
    aspects. | LCSH: Breastfeeding—History. | LCSH: Breastfeeding—
    Political aspects. | LCSH: Breastfeeding—Psychological aspects. |
    LCSH: Breastfeeding—Health aspects. | LCSH: Breastfeeding
    promotion.
Classification: LCC RJ216 .R57 2021 | DDC 649/.33—dc23

Set in 10.5/14 Calluna with Calluna Sans and Neue Haas Unica Pro
Book design & typesetting by Garet Markvoort, zijn digital

For Rosalie, my sister so similar

Contents

Figures

Acknowledgments

To engage in a praxis of humility means recognizing that I'm nothing without the contributions of others to shape who I am. This list will never capture all the people who have contributed indirectly to the creation of this work, including those who may not even be aware of how they changed me.

I'd like to start by thanking Christine Straehle for serving as an invaluable mentor early in the life of the book, reading first drafts, pushing me to just start writing, challenging my thinking about autonomy, liberalism, and care ethics, and always knowing the best places to eat. I'm also grateful for her introducing me to Fiona Robinson, who opened my world to the ethics of care. Another serendipitous experience in carrying out this work led me to meet Emilie Dionne, who has strengthened my understanding of care ethics and theory in general. Thanks also to Shoshana Magnet for reading an early draft, helping me with proposals to publishers, and encouraging me to engage more with intersectionality. Big thanks to Devon Powers for her brilliance and teaching me how to imagine a better future. Jennifer Farquhar Papastergiou provided helpful feedback on chapter 10 and generously allowed me to share her story, although I'm even more grateful for her friendship of almost thirty years. A special thanks, too, to my friend Zelda Abramson, who taught me the value of studying the personal and opened my quantitative brain to qualitative research. I'm not sure I would ever have allowed myself to begin to study breastfeeding if it weren't for Zelda's encouragement.

Endang Purwasari deserves pages of gratitude. I never, ever, ever in a million years would have been able to uncover what I did about Indonesia were it not for her. Before I arrived in Indonesia, she already had interviews lined up, agendas for possible cultural excursions typed out, and all my documents translated. Not only was she fastidious in the work, but she was just such a pleasure to hang out with and so engaged in the ideas I was developing. I think we spent half the time discussing humility, justice, and the meaning of life and the other half laughing our heads off at my cultural faux pas.

I'm also immensely grateful to my coven of warrior women: Willow Scobie, Karine Vanthuyne, and Mireille McLaughlin. Your support, love, honesty, understanding, and wisdom made finishing the book possible despite the dramas that swirled around us. I could not have brewed up a better squad to fight the good fight with. I am also thankful for the wisdom of the healing women in my life, including Marybeth Stanton, Meaghan Harris, Joanne Kealey, Karen Sibbald, Amber Miller, Patti Howd, Annie Luopa, Marlia Biggart, Kyera Lamoureux, Ola Levitin, Amy Eichholz, and Anne Galipeau. You all have kept me on the beam and out of the fray when I just couldn't seem to help myself. A special shout-out to all twelve or so listeners of *The Rippey Sisters Podcast*, especially those who have engaged with us on air or through messages – people like Kathryn Rosenberg, Katrina Olds, Parisa Parsa, Maggie Werner, and Cathy Null, though I'd love you all even if you didn't listen to the podcast (and thank you for giving me a way to shamelessly promote it here).

I am always grateful to my students, who engage with my ideas, keep me on my toes, indulge my never-ending use of breastfeeding examples in class, and suffer my stupid jokes. Particular thanks to Fabiola Aravena, John Paul Nyonator, Shannon Russell-Miller, Laurel Falconi, Chantal Bayard, and Darryn Wellstead, for your contributions to work that is cited directly in this book or on other related projects. I am also forever indebted to my teachers, most especially my long-ago dissertation supervisor and frequent collaborator Mary C. Noonan. Many of the ideas contained within, and my ability to see the beauty of statistics, are a result of conversations with her.

I owe a huge amount of gratitude to the women I interviewed for various projects explored in this book, including the lesbian moms who were my very first qualitative research subjects and, more recently, the mothers and organizational representatives in Jakarta and Yogyakarta, Indonesia. To be willing to open oneself to a stranger for research, particularly on a subject as fraught with judgment as breastfeeding, is a generous gift that should never be taken for granted. I am thankful to each and every one of you.

This book would literally never have come into your hands were it not for the enthusiastic backing of Khadija Coxon and the team at McGill-

Queen's University Press. Khadija is a dream of an editor, supportive and thoughtful, and always willing to answer the most naïve of questions I might have. Thank you for believing in my project and telling me to stop reading and just finish. Thanks as well to the anonymous reviewers of this book, who helped me especially in reworking the final chapter and in clarifying my ideas about humility. Huge thanks to my copyeditor, Alison Jacques, whose attention to detail is unparalleled; having her assigned to my book feels like a product of divine intervention.

Despite all my protestations to the contrary, I am who I am (and this book is what it is) above all because of my late parents, Phyllis and Robert Farley Rippey. I'm grateful for all of their wisdom and that I listened to them in spite of myself. Deep thanks to my Uncle Patrick and Aunt Christine Farley for being surrogate grandparents to my children and for always being on my team. I am also profoundly grateful to my three sons, Max, Jack, and Wyatt, and my two stepchildren, Katya and Finn. You are all miracles to me and teach me far more than I could ever teach you. I thank God every day for gifting me my husband, Joel. He is my muse, my one true love, a strong oak next to my choppier waters, and the one who teaches me how to live in the waiting.

Above and beyond all others is my sister Rosalie, who served as my first book editor, turning my tired rambling drafts into coherent chapters that captured the kapow within. Many of the ideas in this book come from decades of conversation with her and I don't know if I could have ever finished without her enthusiastic labours. I am grateful to have even a little of her brilliance shine on me. This book is for her.

Some of the ideas within this book can also be found in my 2021 book chapter "Recherche du bonheur: Comment l'alimentation du nourrisson est passée d'un acte mondain à un acte moral," in *Des imaginaires aux réalités conjugales et familiales: Perspectives interdisciplinaires et internationales*, edited by Laurence Charton and Chantal Bayard (Quebec: Presses de l'Université du Québec).

Breastfeeding and
the Pursuit of Happiness

1 The Let-Down Reflex

When your baby nurses, nerves in the nipple and areola send a signal to the pituitary to release a hormone called oxytocin. Oxytocin causes those little muscles around the alveoli to squeeze, building milk pressure inside the breast, creating a *milk release* (or *milk ejection reflex* or *let-down*). The tiny ducts yawn open as milk spurts down them. You might feel a tingling in your breasts or shoulder blades, you might feel thirsty or sleepy ... or you might feel nothing at all. In the early weeks, a milk release may be triggered just by thinking about nursing or by hearing a baby (any baby!) cry. Your body wants to breastfeed!

Diane Wiessinger, Diana West, and Teresa Pitman,
The Womanly Art of Breastfeeding

Let down (v.): to lower in position, intensity, strength, or value; to depress; to abase, humble. Also, to disappoint; to fail in supporting, aiding, or justifying (a person, etc.).

Oxford English Dictionary

A number of years ago, a friend shared a diaper ad with me on Facebook, in which a mother breastfed her baby in a restaurant. Knowing about my research on breastfeeding and feminism, this friend would periodically send me stories and posts about mothers fighting for their right to breastfeed. The rational side of my brain was delighted to see the ad. Since most babies on television are fed with a bottle, depicting a breastfed baby in a national campaign normalizes the act, reminding people that breastfeeding is neither dirty nor inappropriate to do in public. At the same time, my knee-jerk reaction was that I wanted to punch my fist through my Facebook feed.

My interest as a sociologist in the feminist implications of breastfeeding began with a feeling of failure. When my first child was ten days old, I switched him from breast to bottle. Determined to do better with my second son, I gobbled up books and websites about breastfeeding, asked for advice before leaving the hospital, engaged the services of public health nurses, took fenugreek supplements, and fed or pumped milk every hour to boost my natural milk supply. Brimming with pride, I was able to exclusively breastfeed him for one heavenly week when he was about six weeks old. One week later, I had to start working again to pay the bills and my milk supply went from barely enough to not enough. I managed to nurse him for four months with some supplemental formula, but then he too was switched to formula.

What began as a search for reassurance that I hadn't doomed my children through these failures evolved into a decade of research into the complex questions that infant feeding poses to feminist theorizing. When my third son was born, his brothers were twelve and fourteen and I was determined to get it right. I knew my child would do fine without it, but I also felt better educated and more prepared to be successful. The dominant explanation for why more mothers don't breastfeed is either that many of them lack understanding of how it works or why it's important or that they don't have enough support from those around them. My own research identified financial insecurity and poor maternity-leave policies as culprits. I figured that I had solved all of these problems. Having moved from the United States to Canada, I held a secure job with a luxurious, fully paid, nine-month maternity leave. I had a loving partner who worked from home and doted on me and the baby. I had access to ample advice and was literally an expert on breastfeeding. This would be my chance to exclusively breastfeed my baby for the full recommended six months and then keep on feeding him until he would self-wean, maybe around two years old. My "good mother" badge was within reach.

Except, just like with my older boys, I was slow to produce milk no matter how hard I tried. I pretended to have a total lack of knowledge about breastfeeding while in the hospital and benefited from almost daily home visits from a midwife. I accessed drop-in lactation clinics around the city and nursed on demand anytime the baby began rooting or looking hungry. After he nursed, I expressed with a breast pump that my amazing midwife had lent to me for free. I used a supplemental nursing system (SNS) to prevent nipple confusion by allowing the baby to latch on at my breast and then sliding a thin tube into the corner of his mouth, attached to a bottle that hung around my neck, filled with the precious limited supply of milk I had expressed. I took my infant to a specialist to check him for tongue-tie, consumed herbal supplements and oatmeal cookies, and started a "milk making" board on Pinterest. In the midst of all these efforts, my husband, Joel, commented that our one-week-old's skin seemed a little orange. I disagreed, thinking he was projecting his own fear – rooted in his experience with my stepdaughter, who had been rushed to the hospital as a newborn to prevent the brain damage that can set in once jaundice takes over. I protested when Joel gently urged me to supplement with formula.

Some researchers challenge the notion that breastfeeding causes jaundice, arguing that the problem is in fact "not-enough breastfeeding" (Soldi et al. 2011). Still, the correlation is clear. The reason is pretty simple: jaundice (a.k.a. hyperbilirubinemia) is caused by a build up of too much bilirubin in the body. Bilirubin is produced in the body as red blood cells break down, are processed by the liver, and are then eliminated through our poop. (Fun fact: it's the bilirubin that makes our poop brown.) If we don't get enough to eat, we can't poop and therefore can't get rid of the bilirubin. For new babies, if breastfeeding isn't going well, they poop less and have no way to get out the bilirubin (Maisels 2015). Some degree of jaundice is common, but if it progresses, the infant can develop kernicterus – a rare cause of cerebral palsy (Maisels 2015). Although kernicterus is exceedingly rare and no reason to fear breastfeeding, it is nearly non-existent in formula-fed babies. According to Maisels (2010), 123 out of the 125 babies in the US Kernicterus Registry (98 per cent) were not exclusively formula fed. Possibly suggesting that the pressure to breastfeed in spite of low milk supply could be leading to an increase in jaundice among newborns, an independent report by QualityWatch found that in the United Kingdom "emergency admissions for jaundice more than doubled over the decade, from 8,186 cases in 2006/07 to 16,491 cases in 2015/16" (Keeble and Kossarova 2017, 7).

Regardless of risk level, Joel began to get tense. He wanted to support me, but the baby needed to eat. At the urging of the midwife we spent an afternoon lying on a quilt in the back yard for some vitamin-D therapy. I couldn't (or wouldn't) see the change in his colour until the midwife became concerned and ordered some blood tests. Before the day was done, she called to advise us to take him directly to the children's hospital, where he was admitted with dangerously high bilirubin levels. For twenty-four hours, our baby was hooked up to wires and tubes while sleeping in a phototherapy bed. He nursed and received supplemental formula and I stayed close by, using a hospital-grade breast pump to extract as much milk as possible. It was not enough. Thankfully, the treatment worked, and we left the next day with free formula samples and the advice to keep feeding and pumping as much as possible. I was able to breastfeed him for six months, supplementing with formula, and I felt like a failure. For the third time out of three, I was a total letdown.

Even though I knew formula supplementation was the best choice for my littlest guy, I was filled with self-blame. I read that obese moms may produce less milk and shamed myself for my weight. Reading that weight and stress can reduce milk supply, I feared I could have exercised and meditated more. I regretted deciding not to take domperidone to increase my milk, even though the US Food and Drug Administration (2018) had published strong warnings about the medication's potential risk of heart attack and death. Research shows that Caesarean delivery can impede breastfeeding, and I had managed an unmedicated vaginal birth with my second child – but the resulting fourth-degree tearing gave me enough pause to choose an "elective" C-section with my third birth. This was also partly chosen after I developed gestational diabetes despite having rigidly adhered to an appropriate diet (my only indulgence was a one-time binge on fresh cherries). This increased the likelihood of a large baby, along with the fact that his brothers came into this world weighing a whopping eleven pounds, ten ounces and nine pounds, eleven ounces, respectively. Avoiding a Caesarean became even more unwise when my blood pressure began to climb and the doctor I was referred to advised that it could be dangerous to allow labour to happen naturally.

It is possible that I could have done something better or differently, but this kind of post-game conjecture implies the problem was my fault. Some breastfeeding advocates might say that I wasn't the letdown, but rather that the system let me down (Allers 2017). As I will argue in this book, this system-blaming evokes what philosopher Lisa Tessman (2010, 798) calls "falsely cheerful" theorizing: suggesting that bad situations are avoidable if everyone does everything right. In reality, sometimes we're lucky and sometimes we're not. Some moms produce tons of milk while others struggle to produce much at all, and this doesn't necessarily reflect how much they want to breastfeed.

There were things I loved about breastfeeding. Among them were the snuggling, the tingling feeling that comes with let-down, and the connection I felt when my breasts would react to my baby's cry. The cost of pads, pump supplies and special clothing seemed preferable to forking over money to a big formula company. And, although I cringe at the argument that breastfeeding is "more natural," it is an ingenious miracle of nature. I mean, how cool is it to be able to sustain the life of another human being with one's own body? I also loved my breasts. They were giant, gorgeous, voluptuous orbs of fullness and delight. Breastfeeding advocates often desexualize breasts to counteract the idea that public breastfeeding is obscene, but I felt lusciously sexy and full of life. My favourite part of breastfeeding, though, was the experience of a hungry baby rooting around, trying to find a nipple. When babies are seeking their sweet nectar, they will shake their heads back and forth almost frantically. Finally, hungrily latching on, they just relax into it, sometimes literally sighing. Some babies grow quiet, and others will paw at their mother with their tiny fingers, pulling gently on her hair. Sometimes a lower arm will wrap around the mother, or their legs will flap and squirm. Easing back into these memories, I am flooded with the warmth of feeling absolutely desired, loved, and needed in a way that no other person has ever conveyed to me.

Not all mothers experience breastfeeding positively, though. In an interview I carried out for a research project on lesbians' experiences as breastfeeding mothers, one participant told me that during the year that she breastfed her second child, she prayed for her doctor to tell her to quit because she felt too guilty to stop on her own. Breastfeeding can occasionally trigger suicidality as a result of "dysphoric milk ejection reflex," which creates a sudden low mood at breastfeeding initiation. Breastfeeding and pumping can trigger traumatic memories among survivors of sexual or physical violence, although the experience can also become an empowering way to reclaim one's body. Even for those who enjoy breastfeeding, an improper latch can lead to the excruciating physical pain of cracked nipples. With my first son, I recall sitting with my breasts exposed, blowing on my nipples, hoping the cool air might provide some relief. When this problem isn't corrected, one's nipples can become so raw they physically begin to tear away from the breast. On the other hand, women who produce too much milk can experience clogged milk ducts, which can lead to mastitis, a painful infection that is accompanied by flu-like exhaustion. Unfortunately, rest is not an option with clogged ducts since the cure is to breastfeed as much as possible.

Given the preponderance of evidence, "breast" is neither always "best" nor always a choice. While many women could breastfeed but do not, there are also many who want to breastfeed but cannot. There are women who never get help and end up switching to bottles, which leaves them devastated. There are those who get immense help and support and never make it work. There are thankfully many, many women who have no problems breastfeeding and love it. Still others do so easily but hate it. Many mothers and babies will thrive but still some won't. Personally, I am grateful for having had the opportunity to experience breastfeeding in moments that were positively luscious and I'm equally grateful to have had access to formula when my babies needed it. Breastfeeding can sustain life, but without formula, some babies will die.

Narrative Framing

Many women's experiences to the contrary, the act of breastfeeding is widely described as universally accessible, wholly positive, essentially natural, and morally good. This means that feeding infants in other ways is framed as a failure, an anomaly, abnormal, or the result of something going wrong. It is the framing of breastfeeding and its alternatives that is the subject of this book. With catchphrases like "breast is best," "breast-feeding is normal," and "formula is risky," the narratives, or stories, told about breastfeeding claim a foundation on science, when in reality they are moral lessons used to influence human behaviour. Narrative analysis is not traditionally the purview of science, and my own training and re-search in quantitative sociology has emphasized material facts that can be measured using statistics. The questions I have been most drawn to have been those in which the facts do not match people's beliefs. Even more fascinating, however, is when the purported facts are based on people's perceptions. Too often, science is assumed to be objective, as that is its foundational goal. But something usually gets missed when we rely too much on data and ignore the stories and emotions that led to the numbers being collected (Laslett 1990).

As social movements scholar Kathleen Rodgers points out, academic research has long overemphasized rationality to the detriment of under-standing the subjective experiences and emotions of social movement actors. Citing Goodwin et al. (2004), she notes, "successful framing is almost always achieved through the strategic use of 'moral emotions', emotions based on values, beliefs or social expectations" (Rodgers 2010, 275). If successful social movement mobilization depends on "moral emo-tions," then the methods used to evoke and understand such emotions would seem rather important. Scholars of social movements have shown that the strategic use of moral emotions takes place through the use of frames, or collective action frames. Building on the work of Goffman (1974), Snow et al. describe frames (or frameworks) as "'schemata of inter-pretation' that enable individuals 'to locate, perceive, identify, and label' occurrences within their life spaces and the world at large. By rendering events of occurrences meaningful, frames function to organize experience and guide action, whether individual or collective" (1986, 464).

Social movements can also reframe their agenda as times change. For example, Saurette and Gordon (2015) studied the rhetorical shift of the anti-abortion movement from an emphasis on protecting "the unborn" to a focus on protecting women from being coerced into abortion. Thus, the movement coopted a feminist framing of women's rights to convince potential supporters that their movement is neither anti-choice nor anti-woman. This was successful in part because feminist organizing has been so successful at making women's rights a moral good. Though many may dispute whether women actually have rights equal to men, no longer is it socially acceptable to challenge that women *should* have equal rights. Saur-ette and Gordon (2015) point out that this is a particularly effective means of bringing people on board to one's social movement. Citing Kahneman (2011), they write, "frames that mimic or piggy back on other pre-existing, widely shared/recognizable frames are often adopted more easily – for our brains tend to be less critical of, and accept more readily, frames (and other phenomen[a]) that already have a common-sensical or normal 'feeling'" (226). In the case of breastfeeding, it feels true to us to say that "breast is best," despite all the instances in which breast is not feasible, desirable, or safe. This is because the framing of breastfeeding is inextricably linked to widely shared narratives around womanhood and mothers.

The Heroes, Victims, and Villains of Breastfeeding

Saurette and Gordon's (2015) research into anti-abortion rhetoric homes in on the way that stories are used by political actors to teach lessons that can influence the populace. Narratives draw on widely shared and recog-nizable frames that "reproduce predictable plots and often rely on recogni-zable stock characters that communicate the basic moral lesson to the audience almost instantaneously" (278). They go on to explain,

It is thus unsurprising that most political narratives are structurally similar to typical Hollywood blockbusters or childhood fairytales. These stories generally revolve around three main characters: the victim who needs to be rescued, the hero who rescues the victim, and the villain who harms the victim and stands in the way of the hero. Given its prevalence, this structure is intuitively recognizable to almost anyone raised in Western culture: the villain represents what the discourse cannot accept; the victim represents the honourable principles that must be protected/rescued from an injustice; and the hero is the device that gives it nobility, honour, emotional resonance or motivation, and moral worth to the political quest. (278)

The narrative power of heroes, victims, and villains can be found throughout breastfeeding promotion, including in the work of the World Health Organization (WHO), public health agencies, and other nongovernmental organizations. For example, in February of 2013, the British organization Save the Children launched a breastfeeding campaign aimed at poor countries with a report titled *Superfood for Babies: How Overcoming Barriers to Breastfeeding Will Save Children's Lives* (Mason, Rawe, and Wright 2013). Like a superhero, breastfeeding was touted as a solution to the problems facing the most innocent of victims: infants in developing countries. The villains of this narrative were formula companies, policy-makers, grandparents, fathers, and healthcare providers who cause or fail to remove barriers to breastfeeding. The heroic efforts of NGOs were presented as "empowering" poor women to make the "right" feeding decisions, but the women themselves were portrayed as victims and not as heroes. For example, the first barrier to successful breastfeeding is "community and cultural pressures"; the report's authors write,

Despite clear evidence that early and exclusive breastfeeding is the best way to care for newborns, many mothers in poor countries are given bad advice or are pressured into harmful alternatives ... Many women are not free to make their own decisions about whether they will breastfeed, or for how long. In Pakistan, a Save the Children survey revealed that only 44% of mothers considered themselves the prime decision-maker over how their children were fed. Instead it is often husbands or mothers-in-law who decide. (viii)

The moral framing of this rhetoric adds persuasive power because it is so familiar. Faced with the problem of infant mortality, we want someone to root for, someone to blame, and someone to feel empathy for. Who wouldn't want to see a world in which babies are saved, women empowered, and the unfairly powerful felled? The problem is that this storyline of heroes, victims, and villains has developed over thousands of years within contexts defined and dominated by powerful men. If it were merely an effective rhetorical device to promote policies that are in the best interests of women and children, perhaps we could let this slide. But the impact of this narrative on women's lives must be considered.

Considering that only 20 per cent of American mothers meet the recommended goal of six months of exclusive breastfeeding, 80 per cent of infant feeding experiences are thus a failure. Although feminist breastfeeding advocates would argue that the system is failing, there is much evidence that individual mothers, myself included, experience this as a personal failing. When I started writing this book, I googled "did not breastfeed." The first result of over three million was, "How do I handle my feelings of failure for not breastfeeding?" A more recent search turned up normalizing yet defensive posts such as "5 Women Explain Why They Chose Not to Breastfeed" and "I didn't breastfeed my children & they turned out great." The meta-description offers, reassuringly, "I felt like I had 'failed' her, and myself, in some way." Clearly, I'm not the only one feeling like a letdown.

Breastfeeding and the Pursuit of Happiness

As we will explore in this book, the feeling that breastfeeding is essential to motherhood didn't come from nowhere. I will show that prescriptions and proscriptions about infant feeding have as much to do with a broader pursuit of happiness as they do with actual concern for the health and well-being of babies and mothers. Historian Darrin McMahon (2006) argues that the pursuit of happiness has been a central preoccupation of Western thought since at least the ancient Greeks. We see traces of this pursuit in the Bible and other religious texts, continuing through seventeenth- and eighteenth-century liberal philosophy and within popular culture today. Building on this observation, feminist scholar Sara Ahmed argues in *The Promise of Happiness* that the discourse of happiness makes an effective tool of oppression:

Feminist critiques of the figure of "the happy housewife," black critiques of the myth of "the happy slave," and queer critiques of the sentimentalization of heterosexuality as "domestic bliss" have taught me most about happiness and the very terms of its appeal. Around these specific critiques are long histories of scholarship and activism which expose the unhappy effects of happiness, teaching us how happiness is used to redescribe social norms as social goods. (2010, 10)

She points to Simone de Beauvoir's assertion, made in 1949, that "there is no possibility of measuring the happiness of others, and it is always easy to describe as happy the situation in which one wishes to place them" (quoted in Ahmed 2010, 10). In other words, systems of domination can be reinforced by suggesting that the oppressed are happy with their lot. In this book, I argue that breastfeeding has proven particularly successful in this regard.

As Ahmed writes in her discussion of Jean-Jacques Rousseau's *Émile*, happiness can be found by following "nature's path" (2010, 80). Disobeying nature's will for us will bring frustration and misery to ourselves and go against the common good. To Rousseau, men need women for society to flourish; "for women to be educated to be anything other than wives for men would hence take them away from nature, and from what can promise happiness" (Ahmed 2010, 80). Interestingly, breastfeeding occupies a great deal of Rousseau's attention in *Émile*, a fact that has not made its way into most contemporary breastfeeding debates (Kukla 2005). I will return to Rousseau in a later chapter, but notable here is that "nature" is never used to examine the natural capacities of men's nipples. All human beings are born with nipples and milk ducts regardless of their assigned or chosen sex, with varying capacities for milk production. However, the idea of fathers' nipples being used to soothe babies has almost never been explored. Transgender men who give birth can chestfeed, but this has sown controversy among some breastfeeding advocates (Tapper 2014). The nipples of those born with male sex organs are typically framed as vestigial or useless outside of the Aka people, a nomadic pygmy tribe from the western Congo Basin who are remarkable for the extent to which parenting responsibilities are shared, including making use of fathers' nipples for nurturing babies (Hewlett 1989).

Given that at least one culture has found a purpose for men's nipples, we can see that framing breastfeeding as a women-only domain is a cultural construction as opposed to a natural or biological fact. We can therefore be skeptical of the claims that breastfeeding is "only natural" and is required for human happiness. Put another way, it seems an unlikely coincidence that the framing of breastfeeding as the sole and rightful domain of women happens to align with patterns of male domination stretching back thousands of years.

I am not the first to point out this connection. Drawing on sociobiological and anthropological evidence, Joan Huber (2007) creates a compelling case that breastfeeding is at the root of gender inequality today because from the dawn of human evolution, it prevented women from engaging in the practices that have allowed men to collect resources and garner power. Though Huber's research explores time periods that predate written history, we know that breastfeeding has been used in written texts to justify women's role in society at least since Aristotle (384–322 BCE). As Papastavrou et al. explain, the philosopher "considered breastfeeding a maternal duty and [was] opposed to the use of wet nurses. He asserted that the quality of food exerted maximum effect in the organism and breast milk was the best food for the babies" (2015, 3). Claims of breast milk's medicinal and healing properties have been associated not just with health but also with happiness. Much as the Bible promises a land of milk and honey for the faithful, Marylynn Salmon (1994) writes of seventeenth-century American colonial ministers who likened the happiness of heaven to the bliss an infant feels at the mother's breast. Thus, although the expression "breast is best" has a trendy ring to it, the moral purity it implies is nothing new.

Liberation or Instruments of Oppression?

While there has been no shortage of men's opinions about breastfeeding throughout Western history, there is an equally long history of women seeking alternatives to mother's milk. With advances in sanitation and industrial food production came the rise of infant formula as capitalists worked in collaboration with the newly expanding medical field of pediatrics, to their mutual profit (Nathoo and Ostry 2009). Whereas breastfeeding advocates are critical of the marketing of formula and the impact this invention has had on global breastfeeding rates, others have pointed to the introduction of formula as an important factor contributing to the rise in women's labour-force participation in the early twentieth century (Albanesi and Olivetti 2016). Sociologist Mary Noonan and I also found that women who breastfeed longer experience steeper earnings losses (Rippeyoung and Noonan 2012b) and lower rates of father involvement in infant care (Rippeyoung and Noonan 2012a). Additionally, in qualitative interviews of lesbian mothers, Laurel Falconi and I found that breastfeeding impacts the division of labour in households, even in the absence of men (Rippey and Falconi 2016). Thus, there are numerous ways which breastfeeding has and continues to reinforce traditional divisions of labour.

It is important to pause for a moment to consider whether women's participation in labour markets should be our goal. In other words, is paid work the goal of feminism, or is it just another tool of oppression? Patricia Hill Collins (2008) and Hazel Carby (2000) both argue that paid labour has brought exploitation to the lives of many women, and particularly to the lives of Black and Indigenous mothers. Collins points to the greater meaning African American women often find in "motherwork" than can be found in paid work within a racist social structure. For those whose paid work or slave labour has torn them away from their children and families, breastfeeding may feel like a privilege and a form of labour to be savoured. The right to breastfeed one's infant is as worthy a freedom to fight for as any other act of women's self-determination. However, the reality of our political and economic system is that women, regardless of race, are not rewarded financially for this domestic work and in fact pay a steep financial penalty for doing what's purportedly "best" for their children and society.

Further, although breastfeeding can be supported through strong maternity-leave policies and economic protections for vulnerable families, too often these policies are dismissed as too expensive, despite breastfeeding being touted as the cure for myriad social problems. Breastfeeding promotion has been a cornerstone of global development programs since the 1970s. Starting with UNICEF and the WHO, breastfeeding has been touted as "the closest thing there is to a 'silver bullet' in the fight against malnutrition and newborn deaths" (Mason, Rawe, and Wright 2013, vii). In 1990 the WHO issued the Innocenti Declaration, which recommended exclusive breastfeeding for six months followed by continued breastfeeding for two years or more. It is a common misconception that these guidelines were strictly based on medical research. Yet a talk by Ted Greiner (2000), former director of the Swedish International Development Agency and internationally recognized breastfeeding advocate, revealed on the anniversary of the Innocenti Declaration that the recommended two years of breastfeeding was a result of pressure by delegates from Muslim countries who insisted on following what is recommended in the Qur'an.

Infant mortality is not the only social problem that breastfeeding has been promised to solve. In 2016, the prestigious British journal *The Lancet* published a series of articles on the benefits of breastfeeding. The series began with an editorial that states,

> Breastmilk makes the world healthier, smarter, and more equal: these are the conclusions of a new Lancet Series on breastfeeding. The deaths of 823 000 children and 20 000 mothers each year could be averted through universal breastfeeding, along with economic savings of US$300 billion. The Series confirms the benefits of breastfeeding in fewer infections, increased intelligence, probable protection against overweight and diabetes, and cancer prevention for mothers. The Series represents the most in-depth analysis done so far into the health and economic benefits that breastfeeding can produce. ("Breastfeeding" 2016, 404)

Upon its publication, the WHO, UNICEF, and other organizations issued press releases with headlines like "New evidence in the Lancet shows more benefits of breastfeeding" (UNICEF 2016; PAHO/WHO 2016). UNICEF chief of nutrition Werner Schultink was quoted as saying, "The Series provides crucial evidence for the case that breastfeeding is a cornerstone of children's survival, health, growth and development and contributes to a more prosperous and sustainable future" (UNICEF 2016). According to all of these sources, this miracle cure for all that ails the world would come to pass if there just weren't so many barriers to ensuring mothers could breastfeed.

Concerns about these barriers are summarized in an article published in the *International Journal of Children's Rights* by the late Michael Latham, a Cornell University nutritionist and breastfeeding advocate. Latham wrote,

> Infants' interests in optimal health and nutrition may be jeopardized if not fed on human breastmilk, or even if not breastfed. This should be viewed in terms of ethical, moral or civic interests and duties, not as legal obligations on the mother deriving from legal rights of the infant. We should help mothers understand the benefits

of breastfeeding to themselves and their infants. We can then agree that states have responsibilities and obligations to respect, protect, support and promote the removal of all obstacles to breastfeeding. When this is achieved, it probably will be unusual for infants not to be breastfed. (1997, 416)

Here Latham is trying to walk a tightrope by asserting the "ethical, moral or civic" duty for babies to be breastfed, while promising that mothers should not be legally obligated to do so. His solution to the potentially competing rights of infants and mothers is to fully inform women of the benefits of breastfeeding and ensure nothing gets in the way. Given the opportunity, Latham insists, women will want to do it. As tidy as this would be, the question remains: What if they don't? If not being breastfed deprives a baby of their natural rights and depresses their future potential, what do we do with the villainous women who refuse or fail to do what's "right" for their babies and for society?

The unsettling juxtaposition of the rights of infants and the rights of their mothers would seem to make breastfeeding a fertile ground for feminist debate. Yet major women's rights organizations have had little to say about infant feeding, and breastfeeding is not a particularly common subject for feminist, critical race, or postcolonial theorizing. Even the groundbreaking booklet *Women and Their Bodies* (precursor to *Our Bodies, Ourselves*) (BWHC 1970), mentioned breastfeeding only in a fleeting few sentences, referring struggling women to the international support group La Leche League (Jacqueline Wolf 2006). This vague treatment of breastfeeding in such a comprehensive resource on women's bodies may have reflected the feminist rejection of maternity as women's destiny. At the same time, feminists of the 1970s did join calls to boycott the multinational corporation Nestlé for exploiting and profiting off of women's vulnerability in low-income countries (Baumslag and Michels 1995). Later, as breastfeeding became increasingly expected of mothers through the 1980s and 1990s, pro-breastfeeding feminists focused on protecting women's breastfeeding rights and arguing that nursing protects the health and well-being of children and mothers. These "maternalist" feminists (Allers 2017; Hausman 2003; Van Esterik 1989) argued that failing to support breastfeeding constrains women's autonomy and deprives them of their rights. In this context, public breastfeeding is framed as a political act in defiance of patriarchal social norms.

Over the past fifteen years or so, new challenges have been raised to the notion that breastfeeding is empowering for women or "best" for babies (Badinter 2010; Barston 2012; Rosin 2009; Joan Wolf 2010). Breastfeeding promotion has been criticized on the basis that promoting one manner of infant feeding constrains women's autonomy to do as they choose with their bodies (Balint, Eriksson, and Torresi 2018; Kukla 2006). Within and across these debates are questions about the role of race and class in breastfeeding advocacy. Lower rates of breastfeeding among Black women than White women have been attributed to racism in the medical field (Freeman 2018; Hausman 2003), the impact of White women's historical exploitation of Black women as wet nurses (Freeman 2018; Roberts [1997] 2014; West and Knight 2017), and current and historical racist portrayals of Black women's bodies as savage, exotic, animalistic, and sexualized (Blum 1999; Freeman 2018).[1]

Interestingly, within breastfeeding debates, many scholars seem to agree that breastfeeding must be understood differently in developing countries than in the West. Even feminists calling for "choice" in infant feeding make an exception for mothers "in the developed world" who may lack access to clean water (see, e.g., Joan Wolf 2010). Drawing a boundary between infant feeding prescriptions for Western women and those for women from developing countries would seem to imply that some women are more entitled to self-determination than others. More concretely, making this concession allows the deeper problems of water access to go unquestioned. In a very real sense, it accepts the sacrifice of women's bodies in lieu of enacting deeper structural change to the oppressive global systems that created unsafe conditions in the first place.

What I will lay out in this book are the ways in which breastfeeding is implicated in the development and maintenance of numerous patriarchal, White supremacist, and exploitative capitalist systems. The exceedingly long history of using infant feeding to control, exploit, and otherwise dominate women contradicts any notion that breastfeeding is simple or a matter of choice. For millennia, breastfeeding rhetoric has transformed infant feeding from a basic human need into a solution for any number of problems, including the pursuit of happiness itself.

What makes breastfeeding such a fertile ground for exploring the oppression and liberation of women is that it taps into the most basic human needs to give and receive care. Being thwarted from taking care of oneself or one's babies is an injustice, but whether the injustice is driven by structures of domination or by one's own body will influence with whom one is to lodge a grievance. Further, the historical record shows that breast-feeding rhetoric has better served the interests of the powerful than the interests of those who perform (or fail to perform) this embodied labour.

Drawing on Black feminist theory (Carby 2000; Collins 2008), postcol-onial feminism (Carby 2000; Mohanty 2003), material feminism (Federici 2014), affect theory (Ahmed 2010), feminist care ethics (F. Robinson 2011; Tronto 2013), and, most explicitly, theories of political humility (Button 2005; Rushing 2020) and Hannah Arendt's *The Human Condition* ([1958] 2018), I propose that the resolution to the question of whether breast-feeding is liberating or oppressive can be found with an ethos centred on care (rather than rights), with action based in humility – what I call a "praxis of humility." The term "praxis" comes from Aristotle, who dis-tinguished *praxis* (action) from *ethos* (morality) (Belfiore 1983). Though *praxis* is also a common theme discussed by Marx and Marxists as a kind of theory-informed practice or behaviour, the concept was revived in the Aristotelian sense by Arendt in her discussion of what comprises the *vita activa* within the human condition. I borrow from her work to conceptual-ize humility as a *praxis*, or an action that one can engage in, rather than as an *ethos* or a moral quality inherent in a person.

Humility is a way of acting that shifts beyond a binary of good and bad to recognize that we all have the capacity to help and to hurt, to give and to receive. Within a praxis of humility, the framework for hero, victim, and villain breaks down, exposing the damage that these narratives cause. I will apply this theory to discourses surrounding infant feeding, including "breast versus bottle debates," which exemplify a lack of humility as each "side" claims to be the hero. Patronizingly dubbed "mommy wars," these arguments increase tensions not only between mothers but also between mothers and child-free women and between genders. Only through hu-mility can we move in a direction where children, mothers, and all others are cared for.

This book will not tell anyone how they should feed their babies. Breast-feeding can be powerful, and were it not for mothers' breastfeeding, none of us would be here. However, there is also power in the ability of scien-tific formulas to feed and sustain babies in a way that makes it possible for birth-givers to share in the labour and love that comes with feeding and sustaining new life. What is clear to me is that concepts such as "best" and "natural" fail to account for how difficult breastfeeding is to do and the oppressive narratives within which it has been framed. To believe un-questioningly that breastfeeding is good can lead to the conclusion that women should be legally mandated to do it, as is the case in the United Arab Emirates and Indonesia. By accepting that breastfeeding is pure and natural, it might follow that women should be able to do it without any help or support. Mired in the debate over whether breast is best or breast-feeding is unworthy of theoretical attention, feminists have been spinning their wheels. Through a praxis of humility, I believe, we can see breast-feeding for what it is: a part of life that is both as mundane as urine and as incredible as the discovery that urine contains enough potential energy to power a cell phone (Kalan 2014). In much the same way, pursuing world happiness through breastfeeding is as likely to yield satisfaction as would a pursuit of happiness through the meaning of our pee.

1   In this book, "Black" and "White" are capitalized to acknowledge the historical and social construction of racial categories (Appiah 2020).

2 Theorizing Breastfeeding

Every day, women who fought for independence and autonomy, are being told which pursuits are worth the sacrifice – which areas of our life are "worth" overcoming challenges for and which are not. There is a popular refrain that breastfeeding is too hard and too difficult for the payoff. We are fed messages that toned bodies are worth hours of sweating in the gym and the cost of buying expensive products to achieve, but somehow contributing to the long-term health of our children is not worth any committed effort. We encourage each other to crash through glass ceilings, use off-ramps and on-ramps to maintain our career and to "lean in" for greater corporate success – but with breastfeeding we are told to give up and not feel bad. And any impassioned support to continue is misconstrued as pressure. That is deeply troubling as a feminist.

Kimberly Seals Allers, *The Big Letdown: How Medicine,
Big Business, and Feminism Undermine Breastfeeding*

In her recent call to arms, *The Big Letdown*, journalist and "infant health advocate" Kimberly Seals Allers (2017) details the multitude of reasons for "how medicine, big business, and feminism undermine breastfeeding," as stated in the book's subtitle. Although her book is a bit fast and loose in the lumping of all feminists into one anti-breastfeeding crew, ignoring nuances of feminist theorizing and many feminist breast-feeding advocates who have been making similar claims for almost twenty years, Allers is right that mainstream feminism has not been able to come to an agreement as to the most "feminist" argument around breastfeeding. There has been minuscule attention by feminist theorists regarding breast-feeding, and there has been increasing polarization between feminists who critique breastfeeding promotion and those in breastfeeding promotion who are critical of feminists. Among feminists, many will advocate for "choice" in infant feeding as a solution to the challenges of breastfeeding, not taking fully into account the structural inequality that makes breastfeeding unjustly difficult. However, many feminist breastfeeding advocates share Allers' concerns and seek to reframe breastfeeding as a social justice issue requiring wider structural change than demanded by the "choice" feminists (Smith 2018).

Like most antifeminist (or one could say a-feminist) breastfeeding advocates, Allers (2017) locates responsibility for the problems surrounding breastfeeding within the control of modern medicine and big business, and, unlike many advocates, she adds "feminists" to her list of those who have let women down in terms of being able to breastfeed. What she refers to as "choice" feminists are those such as Joan Wolf (2010) and Elizabeth Badinter (2010) who dispute the notion that breastfeeding is important at all, refusing to engage with any policy that might emphasize protection of this specifically woman-centred act. Feminist breastfeeding advocates, such as Bernice Hausman (2003) and Penny Van Esterik (1989), have, in some ways, bridged these two approaches by suggesting that breastfeeding should be an important feminist and social goal, and thus we need to break down the barriers to breastfeeding. In fact, they further suggest that in so doing, breastfeeding promotion can dismantle male supremacy by challenging a world order that allocates women's bodies to the private sphere.

However, what all these perspectives seem to miss are the ways in which breastfeeding itself has been used for hundreds, if not thousands, of years to create this system of male dominance. Rather than picking a "side" in these debates, my goal is to transcend them and find a way forward that considers the important insights on all sides while respecting women's lived experiences. In this chapter, I outline the contours of these debates to show that there has yet to be a means of theorizing breastfeeding that doesn't let someone down.

Breastfeeding Advocacy and the Public Sphere

Michael Latham, a nutritionist and breastfeeding advocate, identifies the "lack of community support for mothers to initiate, sustain, and maintain breastfeeding" (1997, 403) as the most significant obstacle women face in exercising their right to breastfeed. He points to La Leche League as almost a refuge from the onslaught of potential threats to breastfeeding within a "non-breastfeeding culture." As he explains,

All too often there are community obstacles to breastfeeding – for example many community women may question the decision of the new mother to breastfeed (and may even be prejudiced against it); many may talk to each other about the disadvantages and potential problems; the community may not approve of breastfeeding in public; the local hospitals and clinics and health facilities may not be supportive, and may not adopt ethical practices related to the promotion of infant formula in their institutions; the work place may make breastfeeding difficult; and there may be no support groups. These and other obstacles to breastfeeding are infringements on the right of mothers to breastfeed. (413)

Latham is not alone in raising concerns about community support for breastfeeding, even if it is somewhat unusual to blame "community women … talk[ing] to each other about the disadvantages and potential problems" of breastfeeding. Most feminist breastfeeding advocates would not argue that mothers' sharing of their negative experiences of breastfeeding is itself an "infringement on the right of mothers to breastfeed." Still, the subject of shaming mothers for breastfeeding in public is an important area of concern for those who view breastfeeding as a right.

In terms of grassroots activism, anger about infringing upon this right has led "lactivists" (Jung 2015) and breastfeeding mothers to stage "nurse-ins" as a means to protest businesses that tell them to cover up (Lane 2014). One example went viral online in 2014, when a mother was denied the right to breastfeed her son in a Victoria's Secret store after she had made $150 worth of purchases. The clerk who refused her request to use a private dressing room suggested instead that she nurse her son in the alley outside (Holohan 2014). The resulting public outcry highlighted the hypocrisy of objectifying and sexualizing breasts while also banning breasts when used for feeding. The national Victoria's Secret corporate office issued a statement of apology at the time, claiming to take the issue very seriously. However, regardless of the company's official policy, another mother, Celina Barbour, was shamed by shoppers at a different Victoria's Secret in 2017 for nursing her four-month-old, whom she was wearing in a baby carrier while browsing the store's goods. Multiple customers gave her dirty looks and one customer asked, "Why would you do that in here?" The experience led Barbour to create a PSA video with her husband, calling out those who feel uncomfortable at the sight of a breastfeeding baby in "a store about boobs" (Levy 2017).

Public breastfeeding has become increasingly trendy, as moms clap back against public shaming, particularly on social media, although there is a double edge to this trend. Bayard (2018) recently analyzed fifty breast-feeding photographs, a.k.a. "brelfies," that celebrities had published on Instagram, noting that breastfeeding advocates have been encouraging mothers to post such pictures as a means to normalize breastfeeding and challenge social media platforms that had previously removed pictures of breastfeeding mothers from their pages. Bayard found that while the photographs were presented to normalize breastfeeding, they also help celebrities develop their brand and sell or market the products with which they are associated. One example is an Instagram photo of plus-size model Tess Holliday breastfeeding her baby while getting made up for a photo shoot with plus-size-clothing retailer Pennington's, where she evokes a similar shot by supermodel Gisele Bündchen from 2013. Bayard quotes Holliday's words in the caption to her pic:

> @nickhollidayco captured this photo of me getting ready yesterday to shoot the next instalment of my #mblmxtess @penningtons collection, and it reminded me of @gisele's iconic photo breastfeeding on set [hand with nail polish emoji] Working moms come in all shapes, sizes, colors & creeds! #normalizebreastfeeding #working-mom #whorunstheworld (cited in Bayard 2018, para. 36)

Thus, Holliday was able to use breastfeeding to build her brand as a good, beautiful, and socially aware working mother.

Though celebrity brelfies may help brand development by signalling "good" motherhood, they also can obscure the reality and messiness of new motherhood. Celebrity mothers appear free of the scars of childbirth, and not shown are their nannies, makeup artists, trainers, personal assistants, and other staff who help them to "have it all." Bayard (2018) thus suggests that by normalizing breastfeeding, such images actually minimize the obstacles to breastfeeding, such as the difficulties in juggling work and new motherhood or the physical pains that can result when mothers don't have the material resources or lactation supports to help them successfully establish breastfeeding.

This usage of breastfeeding to mark good motherhood is not unique to celebrities, either. Geographer Rebecca Lane (2014) found similar patterns following a nurse-in that occurred at a Kentucky Applebee's restaurant in 2007. The incident began when a server asked Holly Joyce to cover up after she had started to feed her seven-month-old at her breast while having dinner with her family. Joyce protested, noting that she didn't have a blanket to cover up with and showing both the manager and the server a copy of the state's breastfeeding law that she carried with her; they nonetheless insisted that she leave the restaurant if she wasn't going to cover up. As Lane explains, "from her car and in tears, she called the lactation consultant at the county health department, who advised Holly to send a letter of complaint to Applebee's corporate headquarters" (196). The company's resolution was to make blankets available at its restaurants so that mothers would have a cover available to them in such situations in the future. News of the incident quickly spread from the local La Leche League, sparking outrage and protests across the United States at the idea that breastfeeding is somehow dirty or inappropriate. Activists were particularly angered by the failure to decouple "the nurturing breast from the sexual breast." A clear example of this was found in remarks by comedian/political commentator Bill Maher, who, Lane wrote, "equated nursing in a restaurant with masturbating in public. Women who nurse in public, contended Maher, are either bad at planning or spotlight-seekers" (206).

Lane (2014) posits that the result of these types of protests falls short of achieving feminist objectives. Such actions tend to base their claims for acceptable public breastfeeding on an emphasis that breastfeeding is the healthiest option for mothers and babies and that most mothers are discrete when breastfeeding. As such, they play into narratives of breastfeeding as the selfless act of "good" mothers. She argues that

> while the defense of public breastfeeding that appeared in media reports and activism following the Holly Joyce incident did indeed work to make breastfeeding a more accepted public activity – in that it at once portrayed mothers as the ultimate nurturers while downplaying the sexuality of breasts – it also tacitly reified constrictive notions of what it means to be a "good mother." It is these idealizations of motherhood – the mother as a nurturer who provides only the best for her child and who performs her motherhood wholly separately from her sexuality – that, when upheld,

make breastfeeding fit into normalized spaces of the public sphere
without causing so much as a ripple of disturbance. Crucial in this
non-transformation of public space is the constant affirmation of a
separation of sexuality from the act of breastfeeding, so that when
the public must subject its gaze to the breastfeeding form, it sees not
a display of lewdness, but an act of nurturing being performed by a
good mother. (196)

Thus, although nurse-ins challenge a sexist and anti-breastfeeding culture that prefers to see breasts in sexy bras than to see them in the mouths
of babes, their impact falls short of unlocking the "emancipatory potential of public space" (Lane 2014, 199). In the Applebee's case, Lane found no
mention by activists that women might breastfeed because they enjoy it,
or because they have the right to take up space. The focus, too often, is on
mothers doing what is considered right or best.

The Feminist Case for Breastfeeding

As the previous section shows, breastfeeding promotion is not necessarily feminist in its approach, goals, or impact. Still, several feminist breastfeeding advocates do frame the act of breastfeeding as a potentially radical
act within the oppressive context of a patriarchal society. Anthropologist
Penny Van Esterik (1989), for example, was an early contemporary feminist breastfeeding advocate who suggested that the creation of a breastfeeding culture would require such a dramatic reorientation of society
that the result would be the dismantling of male supremacy. In this view,
the denial of access to breastfeeding support and the shaming of public
breastfeeding stem from a masculinist conception of a disembodied public
sphere, where messy, leaking bodies are to be left at home (Gatrell 2007).
Thus, whether any mother "chooses" to breastfeed or bottle-feed is beside
the point; rather, feminist breastfeeding advocates argue for a reconceptualization of breastfeeding as a right that should be protected instead of
as an assumed biological imperative. Further, they challenge the misogyny
below the surface of a social structure in which women's feeding "choices"
are so constrained as to hardly be choices at all. In this way, they offer a critique not only of the breast-shaming Bill Mahers of the world but also of
feminists who minimize the importance of breastfeeding to women's autonomy. To these advocates, those feminists who suggest women should

just be freed to choose breast or bottle fail to engage in the persistent and entrenched structural inequalities that make breastfeeding challenging. Feminist breastfeeding advocates have also been critical of non-feminist breastfeeding advocates for promoting the idea that breastfeeding is easy and for failing to adequately grapple with the impacts that poverty, racism, and gendered violence can have on women's ability to reach their own breastfeeding goals (Smith 2018).

The most concentrated work of feminist breastfeeding advocacy is found in North Carolina, through the annual Breastfeeding and Feminism International Conference (formerly called the Breastfeeding and Feminism Symposium), which has worked for over a decade to understand breastfeeding through a feminist lens (Labbok, Smith, and Taylor 2008). Though conference organizers and participants emphasize the health benefits of breastfeeding and are critical of the formula industry, they also take seriously "the realities and constraints that women face when trying to integrate breastfeeding into their lives that are affected by gender, race, and sexuality-based inequities in opportunities, resources, status and power" (Smith 2018, 221).

Though participants make clear the value of breastfeeding for feminist theorizing, many have been frustrated by the relatively minimal feminist uptake of issues surrounding breastfeeding. As feminist medical historian Jacqueline Wolf points out, "unlike obstetric practice ... the value of breastfeeding and the factors that contribute to women's inability to breastfeed have languished as virtual non-issues for feminists" (2006, 397). In an editorial in the *International Breastfeeding Journal*, organizers of the 2008 Breastfeeding and Feminism Symposium in North Carolina wrote,

> Although research on breastfeeding has established that it is a
> maternal and child health imperative, yielding optimal short- and
> long-term health outcomes for both mother and child, breastfeeding
> is not fully recognized as a feminist, women's rights or women's
> reproductive health concern. Most second wave feminist scholar-
> ship and activism has presented breastfeeding as an "option" or a
> "choice" that is generally presented as not very different from for-
> mula feeding. A limited number within the feminist community has
> recognized breastfeeding as a women's health issue or a reproductive
> right. In fact, global support for women's rights generally ignores
> the rights and importance associated with all of women's roles as

mothers, opting instead to concentrate primarily on other important issues such as employment and reproductive freedom. (Labbok,
Smith, and Taylor 2008, 1)

Overall, feminist breastfeeding advocates argue that the fight for breastfeeding is a fight for women to be liberated to use their bodies freely. In this
way, breastfeeding is reframed from a maternal imperative, or something
to be accommodated, to something that should be a normal part of life,
which they see as inherently a feminist cause. As critical literary scholar
Bernice Hausman puts it, we need to shift away from viewing breastfeeding as a public health goal or "over-idealising nursing as a romantic,
nurturant ideal of maternal behavior" and focus instead on breastfeeding
as a maternal practice that recognizes "the reproductive burden women
experience through their bodies" (2004, 278). Thus, to Hausman, by acknowledging breastfeeding as labour with "physical meanings," including
"exhaustion, giving, connectedness, boredom, etc.," we can begin to challenge the ways in which motherhood is constructed to women's detriment
without requiring women to reject their unique capacities as women.

Hausman (2004) goes on to argue that when breastfeeding promotion
challenges the power structures that treat mothers as objects to be dealt
with, rather than subjects with agency, it can force open the public sphere
for mothers. For example, she writes, "The fact that many public spaces
provide little or no provision for the ordinary fulfilment of breastfeeding
practices suggests how breastfeeding is excluded from public life, as well as
how maternal practices more generally are shaped by public space" (279).
She concludes,

Breastfeeding provides a focus that encourages us to see women's
bodies at the centre of the dilemmas of modern societies, as women
are increasingly called to labour in ways that disturb or make
impossible the biosocial practices of maternity. The feminist politics of breastfeeding must be produced, however, as they are not
self-evident in the current global conversations about lactation,
which often position women as the problematic intermediary between a child and its nourishment. Only in the context of such a politics will the tensions between maternalism and feminism become
productive debates over women's rights, women's responsibilities,
and the roles of mothers in the world today. (283)

Not only does breastfeeding offer the grounds upon which to make the case for feminism, but feminism has something to offer breastfeeding advocacy in general, she says. In writing about her experiences with La Leche League, Hausman writes,

> Breastfeeding advocacy, the focus of La Leche League's maternalism, needs to be more feminist, because it needs to acknowledge the political meanings of women's bodies that make it difficult for women to breastfeed or which, in some cases, impel women to continue nursing in difficult situations. And without a feminist approach to the structure of market work and its exclusion of the maternal body, breastfeeding advocates will never be able to do more than argue for breast-pumping breaks at work, a practice which, as Linda Blum so astutely points out, disembodies women as mothers.
>
>   What is not needed is continued sniping about whether organised feminism has been good for mothers or good to mothers. We need not argue about whether organized feminism has thought about mothers at all. (2004, 282)

Though Hausman dismisses critiques of organized feminism as "sniping," Kimberly Seals Allers (2017, 2019), an award-winning journalist, author, breastfeeding advocate, and member of the Black Breastfeeding Caucus steering committee, is unapologetically critical of all feminists, including (or perhaps especially) those in North Carolina. In a recent Op-Ed, she points the finger for Black women's low rates of breastfeeding at the failure of White women in the breastfeeding advocacy movement to decentre themselves. By engaging in White saviourism, she argues, these women, as well as those in La Leche League, have failed to adequately engage with Black communities, with the result that the needs of Black mothers are not being adequately addressed (Allers 2019). Despite her critique of these feminist breastfeeding advocates, she has far worse to say in her book about those she calls "choice" feminists:

> Lately, choice has taken on a concerning meaning in third-wave feminist circles. One of the new iterations of feminism is called "choice feminism." In contrast to political philosophies that explore the ways in which structural inequality limits freedom, choice feminism tells us that every individual is free to choose and that choice is empowering, no matter what the choice is. The result is that the term

"choice" is now employed in feminist debates about everything from the sex industry to marriage and makeup to breastfeeding versus formula feeding. Choice feminism dictates that anytime a woman makes a choice, even if it's to engage in prostitution or pole dancing, is an act of feminism. (2017, 183)

Though her situating sex work as evidence for the weakness of "choice feminism" makes me cringe, I share her view that choice perspectives fail to address wider structures of inequality and oppression. Choice feminism *is* an insufficient solution to the politics of breastfeeding, but the feminist critiques of breastfeeding promotion emerge from decades of feminist movement and theorizing that cannot be swept away as entirely wrong.

The Feminist Case against Breastfeeding Promotion

If the majority of feminists seem to be ignoring breastfeeding, it may be because so much of breastfeeding promotion has relied on particular constructions of the maternal role within a family – a construction anathema to a politics that seeks to liberate women from familial roles that are seen to reinforce women's subordinate status (Hausman 2004). For example, sociologist Linda Blum (1999) points out that one of the leading proponents of breastfeeding, La Leche League, began as a group of White Catholic mothers in suburban Chicago who advocated for a mother-centred parenting in which mothers should ideally stay at home while fathers fulfill their important role as financial providers. Unsurprisingly, feminists were not on board with their cause. In early versions of the feminist Boston Women's Health Book Collective's *Our Bodies, Ourselves*, breastfeeding is mentioned only briefly, and some editions were openly critical of La Leche League's pronatalist position (Blum 1999).

Of greater breast-related interest to the Boston Women's Health Book Collective was the objectification of women as a tool of male dominance. As they wrote in their original, stapled booklet, *Women and Their Bodies: A Course,*

As women, knowledge of our reproductive organs is vital to overcome objectification. We have been ignorant of how our bodies function and this enables males, particularly professionals, to play upon us for money and experiments, and to intimidate us in doctors' offices and clinics of every kind. Once we have some basic information about how our bodies work by talking and learning together and spreading the correct information, we need not be at the total mercy of men who are telling us what we feel when we don't or what we don't feel when we do (it's all in our minds!). (Going together in small groups to doctors to support each other is incredibly helpful to us and works wonders of 'humility' on the minds of many doctors).

The purpose of this paper is then to help us learn more about our own anatomy and physiology, to begin to conquer the ignorance that has crippled us in the past when we have felt we don't know what's happening to us. The information is a weapon without which we cannot begin the collective struggle for control over our own bodies and lives. (BWHC 1970, 9–10)

Part of the collective's argument was that the male medical model of the twentieth century, and before, took women's health out of the hands of women and placed it in the "care" of male doctors. This argument is foundationally identical to the critique lodged by the founders of La Leche League, who asserted that the introduction of formula took away women's power to breastfeed. Yet despite this shared concern about the medical establishment, opinions diverge when it comes to the emancipating potential of maternal roles. Whereas La Leche League and other non-feminist breastfeeding advocates see the family as a site of women's empowerment, early, predominantly White, feminists viewed it as constricting and oppressive. As noted in *Women and Their Bodies*,

With modern birth control, women have the possibility to define ourselves as more than mothers. Even though children give us pleasure, the role of mother is confining alone. Child care does provide women with meaningful lifetime work. What's incredible is that so many women choose it. Why? Part of the reason might lie in the fact that most jobs open to women, particularly uneducated women, are more demanding and less interesting than being a housewife and mother. Another reason is that middle-class women find it hard to do housework and childrearing as well as independent work since the society does not provide childcare centers. But most important is the idea that in our society all women are expected to play this role and their motivation to define themselves differently has been suppressed. (BWHC 1970, 45)

Though this passage is emblematic of much of the mainstream feminism of the 1960s and 1970s, these constructions of housewife and mother are not representative of all mothers' experiences of them. When Betty Friedan ([1963] 2010) sparked the second wave of feminism with *The Feminine Mystique* in 1963 by decrying the limits of housewifery for women's fulfillment, she focused on the troubles of upper-middle-class White women who had gone to college and then languished as housewives, bored and unsatisfied.

As postcolonial and critical race feminist theorists have pointed out, most women do not have the privilege of choosing to exit the labour market and become bored housewives. Black feminist sociologist Patricia Hill Collins (2008) is among those who argue that within our racist economic structure, Black women's paid-labour-market opportunities are too often confined to positions as "mules uh de world," in the words of Zora Neal Hurston's Nanny character in *Their Eyes Were Watching God*. Within this context, the family can serve as a site of reprieve, and domesticity can be understood as a form of resistance against a hostile world. Importantly, this is not the same thing as arguing that women will be liberated if only they can embrace their natural maternal role; Collins points to the exploitation Black women experience as unpaid labourers within their homes, even if this form of exploitation is preferable to the conditions they experience in the paid labour market. Thus, we should be unsurprised by Allers' (2017) critiques of both "choice" feminists and feminist breastfeeding advocates, all of whom have centred their breastfeeding politics through a lens particular to White women.

Given this legacy of feminist movement as seeking to dismantle systems that allocate women to the domestic sphere, we can see why some suggest that breastfeeding promotion is antifeminist (Joan Wolf 2007, 2010) or, more recently, that formula is feminist (Tuteur 2019). In a recent Op-Ed published on Slate.com, retired OB/GYN Amy Tuteur, who blogs as "the Skeptical OB," wrote,

> Until recently, biology was destiny for women. The single biggest issue was women's inability to control their fertility – blighting sexual enjoyment, imposing the tremendous economic hardship of unwanted children, and bringing death to young mothers whose last moments were spent agonizing over what would become of their older children. The pill changed that.
>
> Breastfeeding was *also* biological destiny. It bound women to the home and posed serious health problems for babies of mothers who

couldn't produce enough milk and turned to unsafe supplements. Infant formula changed that.

It is easy to understand how making it difficult for women to access contraception, or even just limiting contraceptive-makers' ability to advertise their product, is an unacceptable way of using women's biology to control them. It seems that it is harder for some people to understand that making it difficult for women to access formula, as well as pressuring them to breastfeed, is equally unacceptable (and for the same reason). It is up to the individual woman to decide whether she wants to use her breasts to feed her baby and whether that is the best choice for her baby and herself. (2019, n.p.)

Tuteur is not the only feminist to actively push back against promoters of breastfeeding. Suzanne Barston (2012), Elizabeth Badinter (2010), and Joan Wolf (2010) are among those who argue that a hyper-focus on the benefits of breastfeeding stigmatizes mothers who cannot successfully engage in the practice and has the potential to cause real harm. For instance, Barston argues that efforts to unsuccessfully breastfeed can result in extended hunger for the child while exacerbating or triggering postpartum depression for the mother. Further, overemphasis on the importance of breastfeeding to child health lays the blame for global problems at mothers' feet, masking underlying social problems that lead to both low breastfeeding rates and high rates of infant mortality and morbidity. Finally, the emphasis on breastfeeding has meant that women who cannot engage in the practice have limited access to accurate health information about safe formula feeding (Frank 2020). The combined impact of these harms leads to the conclusion that although women should be free to choose to breastfeed, active promotion of the practice is coercive and infringes on women's right to bodily autonomy (Balint, Eriksson, and Torresi 2018).

Science Arguments

At the heart of the disjuncture between feminist breastfeeding advocates and "choice" feminists is a disagreement as to how important breastfeeding actually is to child and maternal health. To choice feminists, such as Joan Wolf (2010) and journalist Hannah Rosin (2009), the purported health benefits are overstated and based on weak and often equivocal evidence. They argue that historical, and contemporary, patterns of mis-ogyny, particularly pressures on mothers to engage in "intensive" (Hays 1998) or "total" (Joan Wolf 2010) motherhood, explain more of the pressure to breastfeed than does any actual science.

However, this questioning of the scientific evidence for breastfeeding has triggered vehement objections among breastfeeding advocates. Joan Wolf (2007, 2010, 2013) has become one of the most reviled for daring to write an entire book on the subject, titled *Is Breast Best? Taking on the Breastfeeding Experts and the New High Stakes of Motherhood*. In a later arti-cle exploring the meaning of the backlash to her book, Wolf recounts an instance when one critic of her work emailed Wolf's dean, cc'ing Wolf:

> An anthropologist claimed my research is tantamount to advocating cold fusion and, with extraordinary disregard for basic principles of academic freedom, wrote to the dean of my college asking that I be admonished to cease writing, teaching, or otherwise speaking pub-licly about breastfeeding. She later placed me "in the same category of 'scholars' who deny that the Holocaust happened" and concluded, rather ironically, that "there is absolutely no point in engaging [Wolf] in serious scholarly debate on this topic." (2013, 308)

I may have crossed paths with this same anthropologist when a grant I applied for was rejected in part for "uncritically citing Joan Wolf" – a re-jection that similarly likened Wolf to a Holocaust denier. Like Wolf, I have had a number of other harsh critics when I have gone against the breast-feeding dogma.

In 2015, I received an email from a breastfeeding advocate and writer after I had shared one short comment in a Facebook group of formula-feeding mothers suggesting that the research on the risks of formula were far less clear than advocates would suggest. I was at that time struggling to get published a paper in which I found very clearly that some of the supposed risks of formula were actually spurious. As I will discuss in more detail in chapter 7, formula-fed infants are more likely than breastfed in-fants to be fed complementary foods too early, and these complementary foods make infants sick. The paper was eventually published in the *Journal of Pediatric Gastroenterology and Nutrition*, after the work was rejected by ten other journals. At the time she had emailed me, I was not talking about my paper publicly because I did not want the idea scooped, since it seemed like it would be such a bombshell idea, and because I wanted to be careful not to make false claims if somehow the peer-review process turned up some error I had not thought of. However, my Facebook comment to which she was responding was made in relation to an article a group host had posted suggesting that complementary feeding is not actually problematic. That bothered me because I knew from my own original research that early complementary food introduction can be deadly to babies. So, I made a comment simply saying that I was working on a research paper where the evidence indicated that complementary food is dangerous, far more so than formula. My comment was so insubstantial that I was quite surprised later to find an email in my work inbox saying the following:

> Please check out [*name of her own book*] before finalising your piece about the introduction of foods other than breastmilk.
>
> I am sure you have no desire to do harm to families, and the book may change what you think.
>
> Read the Table of Contents and the Responses pages. See [her website].
>
> There is a lot people do not know about infant formula and breastfeeding – people including yourself if you intend to challenge the considered WHO recommendation of around 6 months and then continue into the second year or more. Microbiologists and epigeneticists and immunologists are coming to the same conclusion as WHO from a variety of different perspectives.
>
> All best wishes,
> [name redacted]

As I'll discuss more in chapter 5, what I believe offended me most about this person's email was that she was relying on a logical fallacy by making an appeal to authority while suggesting that I am simply uninformed. I did buy her book, and downloaded it to my Kobo, but I found it to be a long-winded and annoying polemic, so I never finished it. After some digging, I discovered that her book was self-published. Though this was a rather strange experience that could be chalked up to the dangers of making one's views known on the internet, I would suggest that it also is indicative of the tone of debates that tend to ensue when one challenges the "breast is best" mantra. Hers was not the first email I've received from a breastfeeding promoter inquiring as to the intentions of my research, though it was the first that I saved.

The first time I gave a talk on the economic costs of breastfeeding for women was at a departmental brown-bag seminar, when I was a first-year professor. Not long after beginning my talk, a lactation consultant in attendance joined one of my new colleagues in repeatedly interrupting my presentation to challenge what I said. As an inexperienced and sensitive young scholar, I became defensive and anxious trying to deflect their critiques with my own experiences. When they piped in to say that breastfeeding is easier because you don't have to sanitize bottles, I responded that I didn't sanitize my baby's bottles. The lactation consultant quickly retorted, "Well, it's a good thing your son isn't dead," causing me to burst into tears, much to my own embarrassment. She apologized to me a few years later but remained convinced that bottle-feeding is a threat to infant life and that she could get anyone breastfeeding.

What's most interesting to me, however, is that these were not just attacks on formula or on a bottle-feeding culture but devolved into personal attacks on me and my mothering. There seemed to be such extreme hostility towards what I was doing that all social conventions were thrown out the window, the same as one might do if they were to encounter, for example, a Holocaust denier on a college campus. Further, this attack on a young, woman academic was made by two women who consider themselves to be progressive feminists. To them, I was to be lumped in with the misogynists who suggest women should cover up when breastfeeding in public, with no understanding that there might be progressive, feminist, or other reasons to question breastfeeding promotion aside from prudishness or ignorance. In particular, the fact that their words triggered me to burst into tears points to the significant impact that breastfeeding advocacy can have on one's mental health.

The Emotional Costs of Breastfeeding Promotion

In *Bottled Up*, Suzanne Barston (2012) details the emotional turmoil she experienced as she struggled to breastfeed and made the decision to switch to formula. In her book and its precursor blog, *The Fearless Formula Feeder*, Barston voices support for breastfeeding mothers alongside concern about the ways that breastfeeding advocacy has framed formula feeding as abnormal, unhealthy, or less-than. Barston argues that stigmatizing formula not only is problematic for formula feeders but also undermines support for breastfeeding by triggering a backlash among mothers who don't want to be shamed. This is particularly true when mothers who switch to formula are told by breastfeeding advocates that their reasons for doing so are unfounded. In an online interview, Barston stated,

> I see breastfeeding advocates engaging in online debates with
> mothers who swear that breastfeeding launched them into PPD
> [postpartum depression], telling them that their experiences either
> don't matter or were just plain misinterpreted. This is not okay.
> When a woman has postpartum depression, the focus needs to be
> on getting her well. If breastfeeding is helping her, by all means we
> need to support it and not tell her to quit just because she needs
> Selective Serotonin Reuptake Inhibitors (SSRIs). But on the flip side,
> we need to tell her that it's okay to formula feed. Not "it's okay if
> there is no other option," but rather "it's okay" full stop. And it is.
> Even if breastfeeding does offer incomparable health benefits, the
> studies so far have shown those benefits to be relatively small on an
> individual level for those of us blessed to live with money, resources,
> and healthcare. The risk of having a mother who is incapacitated
> by a severe postpartum mood disorder is not so easy to counteract.
> Childbirth educators and doulas could do wonders in this area –
> they could make it understood to all women, both prenatally and
> postnatally, that whether or not you breastfeed has no bearing on
> your worth as a mother. (in Karraa 2012, n.p.)

There is no clear evidence that struggling to breastfeed causes postpartum depression, although there does appear to be a correlation between them (Pope and Mazmanian 2016). Formula-feeding moms have been shown to experience higher rates of depression, but it has not been established whether this is due to negative breastfeeding experiences or indicates that depressive mothers are more likely to struggle with breastfeeding than non-depressive mothers. Some studies suggest that the hormones responsible for lactation, oxytocin and prolactin, may have mood-improving effects and that breastfeeding decreases cortisol levels, thereby lowering stress and improving sleep. However, again, we don't know if perhaps only some women get the same hormone response from breastfeeding, and perhaps those who don't are more likely to switch to formula (Pope and Mazmanian 2016).

Regardless, many breastfeeding promoters suggest that the benefits of breastfeeding outweigh any costs that might come from an overzealous advocacy of the practice. For instance, Jacqueline Wolf (2006) (no relation to Joan Wolf) offers breastfeeding advocates explicit reassurance that any guilt their activities may cause mothers is an acceptable risk, given the potential harms associated with not breastfeeding. Diane Wiessinger, a lactation consultant active in La Leche League who went on to co-write the eighth edition of La Leche League's handbook *The Womanly Art of Breastfeeding*, goes even further. In an editorial article from 1996, she suggests that health providers need to "watch our language" (Wiessinger 1996, 4) when talking with patients about breastfeeding, to make sure breastfeeding is framed as normal rather than as best and that formula is framed as abnormal and suboptimal. She claims that the "breast is best" discourse unintentionally undermines breastfeeding by making formula seem normal and breastfeeding as better. At one point, she brushes aside potential critiques that this might instill guilt in formula-feeding mothers by stating that mothers don't actually feel guilty for not breastfeeding. Instead, she suggests, when women say they feel guilty or ashamed, they are upset about a lost opportunity. Apparently, the way to address mothers' expressed feelings is just to convince them that their feelings are not what they say they are.

As simple as this sounds, it does not seem to take seriously the depth of feelings of hopelessness, exhaustion, and desperation some women have expressed. For instance, consider the following appeal by a grieving widower, who wrote on Facebook about his wife's death by suicide:

> For all the new moms experiencing low mood or anxiety, please seek help and talk about your feelings. You are Not alone. You are Not a bad mother. Do not EVER feel bad or guilty about not being able to "exclusively breastfeed," even though you may feel the pressure to do so based on posters in maternity wards, brochures in prenatal classes, and teachings at breastfeeding classes. Apparently, the hospitals are designated "baby-friendly" only if they promote exclusive-breastfeeding. I still remember reading a handout upon Flo's discharge from hospital with the line "Breast Milk Should Be the Exclusive Food For the Baby for the First Six Months," I also remember posters on the maternity unit "Breast is Best." While agreeing to the benefits of breast milk, there NEEDS to be an understanding that it is OK to supplement with formula, and that formula is a completely viable option. (Remembering Mother Florence Leung 2017)

Regardless of whether breastfeeding causes, improves, or does nothing for postpartum depression, the dismissive refusal to take seriously the reported experiences of new mothers by suggesting they are misinformed or misguided is a form of gaslighting. The term – recently popularized by Lauren Duca's (2016) editorial in *Teen Vogue* titled "Donald Trump Is Gaslighting America" – refers to *Gaslight*, a 1938 stage play twice later adapted into a film of the same name, in 1940 and 1944, in which an emotionally abusive husband tries to convince his wife that she's crazy by doing things like lowering the gas-powered lights in their home but insisting that they have not dimmed. Duca details the ways in which repeatedly denying reality can manipulate people into believing the gaslighter's opinion, causing them to question the reality of their own experience.

In an almost maddening research article published in the journal *Maternal & Child Nutrition*, Webb Girard et al. (2012) attempt to document the relationship between food insecurity and exclusive breastfeeding attitudes and practices among a sample of food-insecure mothers in urban Kenya. The authors state that a substantial portion of the mothers told them that their own hunger led them to feed their infants supplemental foods out of a fear that either they or their children would suffer from nutritional deficiencies associated with their inability to feed themselves sufficiently. However, the authors repeatedly interpret this as an indicator of maternal "perceptions of insufficient milk" rather than actual milk insufficiency, despite the fact that they "did not formally assess depression, anxiety or self-efficacy using validated indicators nor did we have the capacity to examine potential effects of food insecurity on breast milk quantity or quality or measure interactions between these factors" (209). In other words, they have no way of knowing whether these mothers' self-reported experiences of insufficient milk resulting from hunger were true, but they nonetheless assume that the mothers are wrong. The authors then go on to continue this narrative when they cite "a randomized controlled trial in Guatemala [that showed that maternal] food supplements [led to] significant improved rates of EBF [exclusive breastfeeding] to 4 months among malnourished breastfeeding women" (González-Cossío et al. 1998) as evidence that "across a range of cultural and economic settings, a mother's ability to succeed at EBF may be influenced by her perceptions of the adequacy of her diet" (209). The authors conclude their article with numerous caveats acknowledging the limits of their study and stating that they make an important contribution to the literature by even attempting to discuss the impact of food insecurity on breastfeeding practice. As they conclude,

In this population of urban Kenyan women, food insecurity was associated with poorer attitudes towards EBF, including reduced belief in one's ability to EBF and perceived insufficient milk. These results suggest an urgent need to investigate whether and to what extent food insecurity is undermining optimal breastfeeding patterns because currently, infant feeding counselling and breastfeeding promotion campaigns in this and other resource-poor settings do not usually consider food insecurity. (211)

Though this study does not ignore the role of hunger in maternal experiences of breastfeeding, the authors nonetheless still frame the issue around *perceptions* of hunger, rather than believing the mothers in their study when they say they don't breastfeed because they fear becoming depleted if they do it. Particularly interesting is that the Guatemalan study, in which breastfeeding rates increased when mothers were given supplemental food, is interpreted as evidence for the benefit of changing *perceptions* of food insecurity, not actual food insecurity. In other words, the solution for breastfeeding promotion rests on trying to convince mothers of their capacity to breastfeed if they would just try harder.

Not only do such suggestions smack of gaslighting by undermining women's own perceptions of reality, but they are also often factually untrue. Breasts might not produce enough milk for numerous reasons, ranging from the biological to the social, economic, and cultural. In their comprehensive review of the literature from 1998 to 2008, Thulier and Mercer (2009) found numerous variables that can interfere with extended breastfeeding. They note that though the perception of insufficient milk is likely more common than an actual problem of insufficient milk supply, at least 5 per cent of women are unable "to fully lactate ... related to anatomic breast abnormalities or hormonal aberration" (262). To put that in context, this statistic suggests that of the 3,791,712 registered births in the United States in 2018 (Martin et al. 2019), 189,585 birth mothers could have been physically unable to fully lactate. Or, to put it in another context, according to the US Centers for Disease Control, "there are an estimated 1,046,142 people alive in the United States who were diagnosed with Female Breast Cancer from January 1, 2012 to December 21, 2016 (5-year limited duration prevalence as of January 1, 2017)" (USCS 2020, n.p.), which means that as of 2017, the estimated prevalence of female breast cancers across all ages was 0.64 per cent. The highest prevalence is between the ages of seventy and seventy-nine, at 2.05 per cent. This is not to diminish the significance of breast cancer, but rather to suggest that there is something curious about how we define what counts as a substantial problem.

We can also see the absurdity in dismissing insufficient milk as a non-problem because 5 per cent is atypical. It is unfathomable to think of talking about breast cancer in the way that we talk about insufficient milk supply: well, most women don't get breast cancer, so those who have breast cancer may just be perceiving a lump in their breast. One could counter my argument by saying that we have machines and technologies to diagnose breast cancer, so we can know if the lump a woman feels in her breast is cancerous, whereas we don't have such tools to detect insufficient milk. But that is precisely my point. How does it make sense to answer the question of an unknown prevalence of insufficient milk by saying, well, it's probably not as bad as we think, rather than actually doing something about it? In what other areas of medicine is the cure limited to convincing sufferers that their problem would magically disappear if they just believed in themselves and their body's ability to function perfectly?

Further, such statistics are only estimates of "true" primary milk insufficiency and do not include the much more common *secondary* causes of inadequate milk production (Neifert 2001; Thulier and Mercer 2009). According to pediatrician and parenting expert Marianne Neifert,

> More than 50 years ago, British physician Waller attributed early failure of lactation to unrelieved postpartum breast engorgement, or the inability to establish a free flow of milk after lactogenesis occurs. He estimated that approximately 20% of primiparous mothers experience extreme postpartum breast engorgement, with high milk tension and obstructed milk flow that, if not relieved promptly, results in the rapid cessation of lactation. A bottle-feeding mother provides a readily observable example of how quickly milk-laden breasts undergo involution if not suckled. After abundant milk production begins a few days post partum, the frequency and efficacy of milk removal seems to be the most powerful determinant of the milk volume produced in each breast. When accumulated milk is not removed from the breasts, a chemical inhibitor in residual milk and pressure atrophy of milk-producing alveolar glands result in diminished milk production. Even if maternal production initially is adequate, the breasts soon begin producing less milk if an infant does not extract it effectively.

Thus, inappropriate infant feeding routines that result in ineffect-
ive or incomplete removal of milk soon lead to diminished production. (2001, 208)

She goes on to explain that this process of diminishing supply can begin
when babies are taken from their mothers in hospital so that they can't
feed on demand, when mothers with sore nipples resist nursing because
of pain, or if a mother's work or school interferes with her ability to nurse
on demand or to empty her breasts fully (Neifert 2001). Research has also
shown that breastfeeding difficulty can arise from issues such as obesity,
smoking, Caesarean versus vaginal delivery, working hours and precarious work, social supports, and psychological factors (Thulier and Mercer
2009). The solutions for these issues, however, are often presented simplistically as things that are easily changed if women are just given the
right information. For example, Thulier and Mercer conclude their review
article by suggesting that

health care providers can use this information to better identify
and target those at risk for early breastfeeding cessation, specifically
young, single, less-educated women of low socioeconomic status.
Interventions can be designed that specifically target women in high-
risk groups, for example Hispanic and Black women. Peer counsellor
programs are an excellent example of this type of care. Research studies that focus on exploring ethnic influences can also provide valuable
insights regarding interventions that may improve breastfeeding
duration. Biological variables such as obesity and maternal smoking can be directly influenced by health care professionals. Women
of childbearing age should be counselled regarding weight loss and
smoking cessation. Nurses must convey to women how these health
promotion activities can positively influence future breastfeeding experiences. Other biological variables that influence breastfeeding duration include real or perceived inadequacies in milk supply and the
physical challenges of breastfeeding. Education about the process of
breastfeeding and breast milk production as well as proper management of breastfeeding can help to prevent both real and perceived
inadequacies in milk supplies ... These steps, some of which include
advocating for mothers to breastfeed during the first hour after birth,
encouraging rooming in, and advising women to avoid unnecessary

supplementation for their infants, are interventions that nurses can implement that will help women successfully breastfeed. (2009, 266)

As straightforward as such interventions might sound, they fail to take into account mothers' embodied feelings of struggling to breastfeed. In conditions of extreme poverty, when a mother does produce milk her body (like society, it seems) will defer to the needs of the child by taking vitamins and minerals from itself, the mother's body, to provide them to the child (Brodeur-Doucet 2016).

Milk production can also be suppressed when infants struggle to properly latch onto their mother's breast, resulting in inefficient suckling. This leads to a cascade of problems that begins with pain in the nipple and may culminate in what is euphemistically called "sore nipples," which can involve cracked, bleeding, or blistered nipples. Breastfeeding is also a learned skill, and those who have never done it or observed it closely are often surprised by just how much breast needs to go into the baby's mouth for the child to be able to press on the milk ducts to signal to the mother's brain that her milk needs to let down. Once breastfeeding does get up and running, and once the mother's milk comes in (which can take days for some mothers in normal conditions), the mother has to feed her baby at least every few hours, around the clock, to maintain her supply. If she must work or be away from her child for any period, her milk supply can start to diminish. Though advocates suggest that the solution to this is better breastfeeding "management" (Neifert 2001; Thulier and Mercer 2009), even with adequate support and guidance, not all mothers can or want to engage in this gruelling regimen.

The reality is that breastfeeding takes far more effort and resources than do any other child health initiatives. As Taylor and Wallace point out,

Claims of many genuinely happy breastfeeding mothers notwithstanding, breastfeeding is also a time and labor-intensive activity – made more so by our social arrangements – that "serves to restrict women's autonomy," particularly in the way that our culture understands it (Blum 1993, 292). When a woman is urged by her doctor to breastfeed, she is being asked to enter an intimate and interdependent relationship with another human being, one that subjects her to the possibility of shame and to increased surveillance. (2012, 80)

As rosy and blissful as breastfeeding may be for some mothers, for others it's a living hell. In qualitative research I conducted through interviews with lesbian mothers, one woman described how miserable she felt breastfeeding her second daughter. She voiced immense relief when her child was weaned at one year old:

> When I stopped it was great … It really was … it was immediately …
> it almost was like, "I can just hold you; you can just be cuddled now."
> Not that she wasn't cuddled, but it was like our interactions weren't
> breastfeeding [anymore] … Our whole relationship was just a strug-
> gle of breastfeeding so now we had to form a new relationship as
> [daughter] and mom, and mommy, and not just [daughter] and the
> breast or something. I sort of just felt like the breast. I really was for
> that time. So it was great [to quit]. I got to see her personality more.
> I was communicating more with her because normally the way I
> communicated with her was "Oh, you're crying, have a boob." It was
> like I didn't have to actually interact with her … It was just like "Do
> you want a boob? Ok, here fine." (Rippey and Falconi 2016, 26)

In this way, assuming that all mothers would like to breastfeed if given the chance denies the complex and diverse lived realities of different mothers. Many, many mothers love breastfeeding, but that does not mean that all will or do. This mother was a stay-at-home mom who got support from La Leche League to breastfeed "successfully for a year." Her problem was not that she "failed" to breastfeed; her problem was breastfeeding. What I describe as gaslighting is termed "relabeling" by Taylor and Wallace, who summarize it neatly:

> The relabeling strategy … fails to adequately address the guilty
> feelings of those women who make informed and relatively un-
> encumbered decisions about feeding their babies; although many
> women may lack the information or support to breastfeed success-
> fully, or may be constrained by physical, economic, cultural, or social
> circumstances that make breastfeeding especially difficult or even
> impossible, not all non-breastfeeding mothers are dupes and not all
> reasons for opting for formula stem from these types of constraints.
> (2012, 80)

Breastfeeding is not a responsibility that can be shared among other parties, and this places an unequal burden on mothers in ensuring the health and safety of babies. The belief that mothers would want to breastfeed if only support were available assumes that mothers should be willing to do whatever it takes for their children regardless of the emotional toll, financial resources, or time it might take. Joan Wolf calls this total motherhood: "a moral code in which mothers are exhorted to optimize every dimension of children's lives, beginning in the womb" (2007, 615). Taylor and Wallace illuminate the guilt and shame that surrounds breastfeeding, stating, "This standard of total motherhood also casts children's needs in opposition to the needs of their mothers: 'mothers have wants ... but children have needs' ([Wolf 2012,] 615)" (2012, 85).

Taylor and Wallace are sympathetic to the desire to remove the barriers that might block women from breastfeeding; however, they remain "unconvinced that all of the self-labeled guilt that women feel can be explained away by the strategy of redefining it as an emotional reaction to a culture that is often inhospitable to breastfeeding; certainly some women ought to be angry, but many of them say they just feel guilty" (2012, 79). They go on to discuss the ways in which this guilt is an expression of a deeper level of shame experienced by mothers regardless of how they feed their children. They cite Karen Kedrowski's story in the introduction to her book with Michael Lipscomb (2008) in which she describes feeling "guilt-ridden" for not breastfeeding her first child longer, having been chastised for breastfeeding her eighteen-month-old at her daycare centre. According to Taylor and Wallace, "Kedrowski reports that the incident made her think '*I am a perfectly bad mother* [emphasis added by Taylor and Wallace]. I am damned because I didn't breastfeed my son and I'm damned because I am breastfeeding my daughter'" (in Taylor and Wallace 2012, 84).

In their analysis of online message boards for mothers, Taylor and Wallace (2012) found that evidence of feeling like a bad mother, a failure as a mother, or even a failure as a woman was rampant among mothers who fed formula to their babies. They reflect, "In all of these cases, the mothers' emotions go beyond guilt, or the feeling that a particular action, or lack thereof, has broken a rule and caused harm. Rather, they judge themselves as deficient: bad mothers, failures" (85). They suggest that this indicates that the mothers experienced shame rather than guilt, leading to "negative global self-assessments" (91).

Taylor and Wallace (2012) situate their analysis in psychology and moral philosophy, exploring the ways in which shame is far more damaging than guilt. They cite research showing that guilt can lead to behaviour change, but shame is more likely to lead to self-blame; then, in search of relief from self-condemnation, it leads to anger at the ones doing the shaming. Among their conclusions, Taylor and Wallace note that even if guilt can at times be persuasive, there is a strategic disincentive for breastfeeding advocates to engage in shaming, as it may backfire by making potential allies into enemies.

Developing a Maternal Self

Since the early twentieth-century writings of Charles Cooley ([1902] 2017) and George Herbert Mead ([1934] 2015), and later, Erving Goffman (1969), sociologists have come to understand that the self only exists in relation to others. As Immergut and Kaufman write,

> For Mead, the self is undoubtedly a socially constructed and even interdependent entity. The self cannot exist on its own; to have a self requires that one has an attachment to others and that one's sense of self arises out of that attachment. The reflexive impulse, the ability to see oneself as part of others, is a necessary component of the Median [sic] self. If we do not fully internalize the attitudes of others then we are not complete selves. Implicit in Mead's explication is a clear, albeit symbiotic, distinction between self and other. By referencing the self, one is, by the same token, referencing the other. (2014, 268)

Thus, to sociologists, there is no atomistic self, but rather we are constituted, in the words of Cooley ([1902] 2017, 184), as a "looking-glass self" in which we understand ourselves in terms of how we imagine others are seeing us. Immergut and Kaufman go on to note that "whether this is an imaginary or accurate perception, the composition of a self hinges upon there being an other that gazes at us in positive or negative ways" (268).

Considering that only about 20 per cent of American mothers breastfeed exclusively for six months as recommended, the vast majority of American mothers are being gazed upon in a negative way through breastfeeding promotion that suggests formula is not good enough and may even be harmful for infants. (I will return to the alleged risks of formula in a later chapter.) Those women who do manage to follow the rules by breastfeeding successfully for longer than one year are not spared from this negative gaze as they may be accused of abusing their children or behaving inappropriately by breastfeeding for too long (Eslami-Shahrbabaki, Barfeh, and Eslami-Shahrbabaki 2015).

If one's sense of self is formed in relation to others and all infant feeding practices are somehow wrong, mothers' identities inevitably develop with a fundamental sense that they have done something wrong for which they need to apologize, atone, or forever compensate. Given the power and authority of public health agencies and the state to determine what is "right," and given how hard breastfeeding can be, and given the fact that infant feeding choices are among the first decisions new mothers make, breastfeeding is a particularly significant factor in the personal and cultural construction of motherhood, mothers, and by extension, women.

All "sides" of the feminist debate are right. Breastfeeding is an embodied biological practice unique to those born with female bodies and is also a highly culturally, politically, and economically circumscribed activity. There is abundant evidence that women have been denied the ability to use their bodies to breastfeed freely throughout cultures, spaces, and points in time and that the pressure to breastfeed has been used as a justification for keeping women out of public life. Breastfeeding can be both a liberating expression of what it is to be a woman for some and an oppressive, physically painful, and alienating experience for others. As such, the struggle feminists have faced in offering a unified or coherent perspective on breastfeeding makes sense. Given this, I suggest that understanding the history, and not only the biology, of breastfeeding is necessary for addressing this feminist divide.

3 The Search for Milk and Honey

Then the Lord said, "I have observed the misery of my people who are in Egypt; I have heard their cry on account of their taskmasters. Indeed, I know their sufferings, and I have come down to deliver them from the Egyptians, and to bring them up out of that land to a good and broad land, a land flowing with milk and honey."

Exodus 3:7–8 (New Revised Standard Version)

In her book *Lactivism*, political scientist Courtney Jung (2015) explores the reasons why Christians are among the most forceful breastfeeding advocates today. According to Jung, the Bible mentions breastfeeding twenty-five times, and Christians tend to encourage breastfeeding on the grounds of godliness, regardless of any health benefits. Across Christian organizations and parenting websites, breastfeeding is framed as "integral to God's plan for how we are to live our lives" (68). Failure to breastfeed is therefore in violation of God's plan and the use of formula is tantamount to a sin. Interestingly, although breastfeeding is valorized within many religious traditions, there is little textual evidence in such texts as the Bible, the Torah, and the Qur'an for the idea that not breastfeeding goes against God's will.

In this chapter, I will explore the ways in which religious traditions around breastfeeding are less about prescriptions for how mothers should feed their infants and are better understood as a rhetorical device, describing our hopes for happiness, health, and liberation from the perils of life. The power of this rhetorical device, however, becomes uniquely insidious when veneration of women is used as a means to oppress them. Although some may find religious writings irrelevant today, religious narratives retain significant force in shaping the Western imagination (Jones 2001) and can be particularly difficult to challenge as they can be taken for granted as natural, appealing, divinely driven, or simply just how things are.

A Land of Milk and Honey?

The epigraph to this chapter refers to one of the most culturally influential phrases in the Old Testament/Hebrew Bible, which promises deliverance from misery to "a land of milk and honey." This precise phrase appears in multiple books of the Bible, including Exodus, Leviticus, Deuteronomy, Numbers, Joshua, Jeremiah, Ezekiel, Joel, and Job, with numerous other references to milk and/or honey elsewhere, although it is not found at all in the Christian New Testament (Derrett 1984). Some presume the phrase refers to an actual geographic place (Ron and Timothy 2013), while others envision a metaphorical Eden (Jones 2001). Its first mention can be found in the book of Exodus.

For those not familiar with it, the book of Exodus tells the story of how the Israelites were freed from slavery and deprivation in Egypt. As retold on the Jewish holiday of Passover, Egypt's Pharaoh had become alarmed at the growth of the Israelite community in his country and decided to enslave them, additionally demanding that all Jewish male babies be murdered. One baby, Moses, is saved by his mother, who sets him in a basket of reeds and sends him down a river to safety. After a direct encounter with God, Moses returns to Egypt to demand freedom for his people. God sends plagues including locusts, lice, boils, cattle disease, and an angel of death who kills firstborn Egyptian children. When Pharaoh finally relents, Moses leads his people on a forty-year journey through the desert and on to the Promised Land.

The Israelites arrive in Canaan, an area that falls somewhere around modern-day Israel/Palestine, although the precise Biblical location is disputed. The land is described as lush, full of vegetation and grazing lands for cattle, and abundant in game such as goats, birds, and fish (Golden 2009). Given this rich description, it is understandable that many assume "the land of milk and honey" refers to a geographic place with fertile soil and abundant resources. The "land of milk and honey" promise has even become a contemporary marketing strategy for drawing tourists into Jerusalem gift shops (Ron and Timothy 2013).

There is a lot of scholarly debate over exactly what kind of milk and/or honey was on offer in ancient Israel. Derrett (1984) notes that in rabbinic law and the Talmud, milk often refers to goat milk, and honey is the wine or juice of fruits. As he explains, "To the rabbis the promised land bears fruits which produce the flows referred to, either directly, or via the

goats" (181). While some have argued that the honey refers to a syrup con-
cocted from figs, dates, grapes, or carob, given the dearth of evidence of
beekeeping in ancient Israel, Forti (2006) disputes this. She argues that
although there may have been no apiculture in Canaan, the extent of Biblical usage of honey to frame various sayings and admonitions suggests
that ancient Israel was likely rich with wild bees. Further, according to
Cohen (n.d.), honey was an important part of Egyptian rituals, especially
for royals.

There is some dispute as to whether the phrase refers to milk at all. Biblical scholar Idan Dershowitz (2010) challenges this translation of the text,
arguing that the phrase should read "a land flowing with fat and honey."
Ancient Hebrew lacks vowels, and therefore the word *ḥālāb* (milk) may be
a misreading of the word *ḥēleb*, meaning animal fat or suet, he says. Dershowitz argues that if the phrase is intended to evoke a rich and fertile
land, "fat is the epitome of richness, and a 'fatty' land can be nothing if
not bountiful. Indeed, whereas land is nowhere else described as 'milky,'
the Bible is replete with images of an oleaginous land" (173). He further
points to a lack of evidence "that Israelites were uniquely partial to dairy
products." As intriguing as his theory is, he undermines his own argument
when he writes, "That *ḥēleb* is described as 'flowing' should come as no
surprise. The idiom is poetic in nature, and an image of a land flowing
with animal fat in its (heated) liquid state is no more or less fanciful than
a land flowing with honey, or oil streaming from a rock" (174). To my ear,
as someone who has experienced an oil burn, the notion of a land flowing
with hot animal fat sounds more diabolical than heavenly. I also cannot
imagine how the horrifying image of land flowing with molten suet, pop-
ping and sizzling at the first drop of rain, would inspire the Israelites to
follow Moses out of Egypt, honey or no honey.

Regardless of the precise foods we're talking about, it seems clear that
"the statement 'a land flowing with milk and honey' was meant as an important religious statement, as its very repetition bears out" (Stern 1992,
555). However, the exact meaning of the symbolism is as much in contention as the foodstuffs in question. For instance, Philip D. Stern argues that
the phrase reflects a metaphorical rejection of the fertility god Baal (sometimes referred to as Lord of rain and dew) in favour of the Israelite YHWH,
"a living god, who can reliably furnish the land ... with streams of milk
and honey, i.e. fertility and abundance" (555). Therefore, he continues, this
expression "should not be viewed as stereotyped or as a lesson in simple

pastoral economics, but as evidence of struggle" between competing cultural and religious traditions (556).

Where Stern sees a metaphor of abundance, Etan Levine (2000) makes the case that it is a reminder of human vulnerability and dependence on God, given that the most suitable places to produce milk and honey are untamed lands where cultivated farming is impractical. Milk-producing animals require grazing land and would destroy cultivated vineyards and gardens, Levine points out. Therefore, the phrase "land of milk and honey" should be understood as a reminder that God has the power to return the Israelites to a state of wilderness if they break their covenant with God. Why would the Israelites follow the strict laws of their covenant with God if they were promised eternal abundance no matter what they did? Instead, Levine proposes that the word "*zb*," which is commonly translated as "flowing," should more accurately be understood as "'exuding' or 'oozing' ... conveying not a torrent but a steady supply." Therefore, he writes, "the 'land oozing milk and honey' would provide *conditional* survival, not *unconditional* affluence" (56; emphasis added).

Given this, I would actually hazard that basing the metaphor on a real land full of cow or goat milk, liquefied animal fat, some kind of fruit juice, a syrup concoction, or the honey of tame or wild bees would seem rather hollow when compared with the fertile abundance of a lactating mother offering both comfort and, as twentieth-century psychodynamic psychologist Melanie Klein (1957) argued in her object relations theory, a threat of being taken away. A mother's milk can be said to flow from the nipple when her body is producing enough supply, but it actually oozes or is exuded during the first days of breastfeeding, when breasts produce a substance called colostrum. In fact, colostrum looks remarkably similar to honey and has been referred to as "liquid gold" because it is so rich in nutrients.

In his exploration of "milk and honey" in Scripture, poet and essayist Jonathan Cohen remarks that "what ultimately emerges is a startling image whose core is pantheistic and sexual, as well as both sacred and profane" (n.d., para. 4). He transliterates the Hebrew, as "'e-retz za-vat ha-lav oo–d'vash'; literally, *land* (e-retz) *flowing with* (za-vat) *milk* (ha-lav) *and* (oo–) *honey* (d'vash). The word translated as 'flowing' comes from the verb 'zoov' which means to flow or gush," he says (para. 7). While the debate between "flowing," gushing," and "oozing" could be attributed solely to the unique linguistic structure of ancient Hebrew, it seems equally likely that the word choice was intentional – knowingly evoking the potential of the lactating breast to variously ooze, exude, flow, or gush.

For his part, Cohen suggests that this flow or gushing refers more generally to "the bodily fluids issued from the genitals of either a woman or a man" (n.d., para. 7). I can sort of agree, in the sense that our various bodily fluids do behave similarly when exiting the body. Then again, if I put myself into the mind of an Israelite fleeing persecution and enslavement by the Pharaoh but uncertain about trusting this Moses guy who wants to head off in the direction of barren wilderness, I'm pretty sure I would be less reassured by images of land gushing with pee and semen than by those of a place flowing with mother's milk.

Cohen is not actually seeking to be so literal. He is simply making the case that milk and honey are symbolic of fertility, not only in the Bible but in many ancient writings. As he explains,

> In all the earliest cultures in the Middle East, honey was viewed as a gift of divine origin. The ancient Semites attributed its presence to Astarte – the goddess of sexuality, fertility, maternity, love and war – who was more widely revered among them than any other Babylonian god; and this earth mother had provided them with it long before Jehovah appeared. Milk and honey as symbols of fertility appear in the most ancient writings, and the well-recognized cross-pollination of these early cultures perpetuated them. Each one assimilated them, as in the Bible, where the land's fertility is likened to human fertility and sexuality. (n.d., paras. 17–18)

Clearly the Biblical image of milk and honey has its roots in the most basic survival needs. It is not merely sensuous but very sensual, as in the erotic love poetry of Song of Solomon, where the fertility figure of milk and honey suggests the paradise of a woman's body. By extension, a land flowing with milk and honey becomes metaphoric of a divine female figure (Cohen n.d.). Interestingly, Astarte, the Goddess of Love, is the female counterpart to Baal in the Babylonian Talmud (Jastrow and Barton n.d.) – the god argued by Stern (1992) to be YHWH's chief competitor among gods one might pray to in the pursuit of lush and fertile lands. For me, this raises a question: Who among these male and female gods should have dominion over women's lush and fertile bodies?

Another scholar, Athalya Brenner (1999), follows a similarly bodily line of thought in her textual analysis of the role of gender in the Biblical Scripture Song of Songs. Within this text, "associations with [date] honey ... and honeycomb ... are exclusively [female], as is the pairing off of 'milk and honey.' These terms are specific of the seduction scene of 4:9–5:1: the female is the food substances, the male eats them or desires/intends to" (108). Themes of gender, food, and sexuality can be found throughout Biblical writings, Brenner states:

> M[ale] is sweet, in an unspecified manner or as a sweet fruit (once) or a good wine. But F[emale] is much more than that: she is food, she is a food production location. When she is "sweet," she is not only fruit but also and specifically "honey." She is milk and honey, and wheat, and pomegranate, and a garden/orchard, and wine and juice, and a vineyard, and grape-derived dry fruit. She flows with the produce of the Promised Land, with milk and honey and wine and pomegranates (and oils, which both genders share): she is the Land, the cultivated land, the Promised Land. (109)

If we accept, at least in theory, that the terms "milk" and "honey" are referencing lactation, the metaphorical usage of them in the Bible becomes even more interesting. For example, in a detailed exploration of the wide and varying usage of honey and bees in the Bible, Forti uncovers that honey is used as a metaphor for wisdom, healing, overindulgence, and sexual temptation and is used to express "the ideational antithesis between the pleasant words of the wise and the evil stratagems of the Wicked" (2006, 339). Interestingly, these metaphors are similar to depictions of breasts and breastfeeding. Today, babies who are breastfed are said to be healthier, to have higher IQs and lower rates of obesity, and, though there remains great public disagreement over whether a lactating breast loses its sexual meaning, the breastfeeding mother is seen as more virtuous than her formula-feeding peers.

A Twentieth-Century Exodus

The legacy of the Exodus story and metaphor of milk and honey can be traced through many modern works of art and fiction, but one that particularly speaks to these themes is John Steinbeck's (1939) *The Grapes of Wrath*. This Depression-era novel follows the Joads, a family of "Okies" who flee the Oklahoma dust bowl for greener pastures in California, facing a harrowing journey and ending up more destitute than when they began. According to literary scholar Ken Eckert, the novel – despite winning the

Pulitzer Prize for fiction in 1940 – has been variously accused of being sentimental Marxist activism, unoriginal, inaccurate, misleading, "watered-down Christian theology via its failed preacher, Jim Casy" (2009, 340), and only enjoyable to non-intellectual liberals. It has also been likened to the Biblical story of Exodus because its protagonists seek to escape a harsh and unforgiving place in search of a Promised Land.

Open to debate is whether the Joad family reaches this Promised Land. Noting that the book ends with the family worse off in every way, Eckert argues that it should be understood "as an inversion of the Old Testament narrative – if California is read not as a promised land but actually as Egypt" (2009, 341). By the end of the book the Joads have nothing and are living in a boxcar camp. Their one asset, a truck, is flooded by the rising tide of a river that breaks through the levee they had tried to erect. The eldest daughter, Rose of Sharon (not coincidentally a flower referenced in Song of Solomon), labours to deliver what will be a stillborn baby. Unlike Moses, the baby is dead when they send him down river in a little box. The flood rises to the door, and then across the floor of their boxcar, forcing the family out with no more food. Making their way through the flood waters to higher land along a highway, they spot a barn through the rain. Nearly dragging the exhausted Rose of Sharon inside, they find a little boy and his starving father. The boy cries, "He's dyin', I tell you! He's starvin' to death, I tell you," which leads Ma and Rose of Sharon to look "deep into each other." Rose of Sharon asks everyone else to leave the barn, and Steinbeck ends the book with this final paragraph:

> For a minute Rose of Sharon sat still in the whispering barn. Then
> she hoisted her tired body up and drew the comfort about her. She
> moved slowly to the corner and stood looking down at the wasted
> face, into the wide, frightened eyes. Then slowly she lay down beside
> him. He shook his head slowly from side to side. Rose of Sharon
> loosened one side of the blanket and bared her breast. "You got to,"
> she said. She squirmed closer and pulled his head close. "There!" she
> said. "There." Her hand moved behind his head and supported it.
> Her fingers moved gently in his hair. She looked up and across the
> barn, and her lips came together and smiled mysteriously.

In Eckert's reading, this total loss, followed by a "simple act of everyday love" (2009, 354) underscores the novel's structure as an inverted Exodus in which the Joads have left a Promised Land for a place "closer to the bondage of Egypt" (355). Eckert refers to the paradox created by the tragic context of this final scene, writing that "even having nothing, Rose of Sharon 'smile[s] mysteriously' as she experiences the feeling of being blessed. The Greek original of blessed, *Makarios*, suggests an emotion of joy as well as spiritual contentment. Here, significantly, the nadir of physical circumstances finally permits her bliss as she has learned to fully love her neighbor as herself" (356–7). According to Eckert, "Steinbeck himself underplayed the ending in his letters, stating that it 'must be quick' and that there is no 'fruity climax'" (354), but, given that he fought against publisher demands to change it, the scene was clearly important to the author.

Where Eckert sees an inverted Exodus, however, I find a complex, yet fully realized Exodus in which the Joads have indeed reached their Promised Land. As historian Darrin McMahon (2006) argues, the central metaphor of the Exodus story is movement in search of happiness that lies always on the horizon, never to be found. He points out that once the Israelites arrive in their Promised Land, they grow lax in their commitment to God's laws, "resorting to enmity, unkindness to strangers, the worship of idols, and other sins (Judges 3:7). Milk and honey, consequently, do not flow. Spatially, God's people have arrived in the promised land, but morally and temporally, their destination remains on the horizon" (79).

Given Steinbeck's leftist politics, the work can be understood as an allegorical warning against the excesses of capitalism, which reified accumulation and brought on the Great Depression. In a material sense, the Joads experience the exact opposite of what capitalism may have seemed to promise. Yet when Rose of Sharon saves the old man, a stranger, she transforms into a "Mary and even a Christ-figure" (Eckert 2009, 354). Her mysterious smile hints at transcendence as she rescues the man with the nourishing, healing power of the generous maternal breast. Not to put too fine of a point on it, but the birth took place merely hours before – and it was too soon for her milk to have come in. Therefore, in reality, she would have been offering the starving man colostrum, the liquid gold that resembles honey.

Divine Healing at the Breast

This portrayal of a promised land to be found in a mystical mother offering divine healing at the breast is not original to Steinbeck nor unique to Judaism but is an image found throughout Christian history. Marylynn Salmon

writes of seventeenth-century American colonial ministers who likened
the happiness of heaven to the bliss an infant feels at the mother's breast
(1994, 252). Historian Londa Schiebinger explains,

> In the Christian world, milk had been seen as providing sustenance – for both body and spirit. Throughout the Middle Ages, the faithful cherished vials of the Virgin's milk as a healing balm, a symbol of mercy, an eternal mystery. As Marina Warner (1985) has pointed out, the Virgin Mary endured none of the bodily pleasures and pains associated with childbearing (menstruation, sexual intercourse, pregnancy, or labor) except for suckling. The tender Madonna suckled the infant Jesus both as his historical mother and as the metaphysical image of the nourishing Mother Church. During the twelfth century, maternal imagery – especially suckling and nurturing – extended also to church fathers. Abbots and prelates were encouraged to "mother" the souls in their charge, to expose their breasts and let their bosoms expand with the milk of consolation. Even the full breasts of God the Father were said to be milked by the Holy Spirit into the cup of the Son of God. (1993, 398)

Such metaphors are also found in the history of Islam. For example,
Muslim saint and Sufi mystic Rabia of Basra (circa 717–801) wrote of the
divine breast in her poetry:

> I hear talk about the famous.
> I hear talk about different cities.
>
> The most intimate events of families come to my ears.
> I hear about temples and
> mosques and
> saints.
>
> All that can be said I have heard.
> All that can be wanted I
> have seen.
>
> My interest in this world has waned, though
> not because I am
> depressed.

A fish in a bowl I was
a bottom feeder,

but now I nurse
upon a breast
in the
sky. (in Ladinsky 2002, 24)

Like Steinbeck's morality tale, Rabia's portrayal of a mystical truth rejects the excesses of human pride and greed, when she suggests that she is no longer interested in famous people, religious institutions, or other man-made marvels. She now rejects this past behaviour as being akin to that of a bottom-feeding fish, sucking up the slimy crumbs dropped by others. Instead, she "nurses upon a breast in the sky." This ethereal, mystical image of the disembodied mother's breast serves as a symbolic connection to God, transcending earthly and vain desires.

And, although Dershowitz (2010) was quoted above as stating that "land is nowhere else described as 'milky,'" in arguing for his theory of a land of *fat* and honey, there are places in the sky that are referred to as milky, most notably the Milky Way. According to Iavazzo et al. (2009), the word "galaxy" comes from the Greek word for milk, γάλα ("galaxy" in Greek is γαλαξίας). Our galaxy the Milky Way, so full of stars at night as to resemble a stream of milk, was said to come from the Greek goddess Hera. As the story goes, she gushed milk into the sky after casting Hercules aside, either for biting her nipple (Iavazzo et al. 2009) or because he, a half-mortal child, was unknowingly put to her breast while she slept (Papastavrou et al. 2015).

The Ancient Bared Breast

The bared breast emerges elsewhere in ancient literature as a metaphoric transmitter of the Divine. Admiel Kosman (2004) explores a curious example of this, found within the Babylonian Talmud. In this story, two rabbis get into an argument over purity laws that devolves into Rabbi Ahadboi mocking Rabbi Sheshet for his ideas. Rabbi Sheshet becomes angry and in retribution somehow causes Rabbi Ahadboi to lose his ability to speak. Rabbi Ahadboi's mother rushes into the *Beit Midrash*, ignoring the proscription against women entering the sacred study hall. She yells at Sheshet to forgive her son, but he ignores her until she bares her breasts and says, "Behold these breasts from which you have sucked!" (297). Sheshet then prays for Ahadboi and cures him of his muteness.

Kosman argues that the "key to understanding this enigmatic narrative seemingly is to be found in the motif of the male mouth and its relationship with the breast" (2004, 297). In one way, the male mouth refers to speaking "the word of God in its Oral Law formulation" (300). Thus, the flapping of gums by the rabbis in their personal dispute that led to the muteness of one was not to be resolved with more gum flapping but only by the "astounding act of uncovering the breasts (or, in other words: uncovering her heart)" (301). But, why did this brazen act work? In other words, why wouldn't Sheshet have been like, "What are you doing?" and then chased Ahadboi's mother out of the *Beit Midrash*? Kosman offers a few possible explanations. For one, this could be seen as a desperate act that shocked Sheshet into remembering that they were letting their passions take hold of their ability to interpret God's word. By baring her breasts, the mother was saying the men were both no better than suckling babies, if they were going to engage in such infantile bickering; Sheshet's petty behaviour did not reflect the intellectual and cultural authority of a religious scholar. Kosman suggests that the mother's purpose may have been to urge them towards their rightful place of authority – or, by entering a space reserved for men, she may have been challenging the value of male authority.

A third possibility Kosman (2004) names is that the mother's bared breasts would have evoked archetypal religious symbolism wherein the breasts represent the Torah itself. He cites Joel 2:16, which reads, "Gather the people, bid the congregation purify themselves, bring together the old, gather the babes and the sucklings at the breast." He then writes,

> The symbol of nursing now appears in another sense: as a common metaphor for the uninterrupted transmission of the Oral Law over the course of time. Thus, the Midrash compares Moses and Aaron to a woman with breasts who nurses the Rabbis. According to this Midrashic picture, the initial state of Torah scholars is indeed that of the suckling infant, who is nourished by the "mother's milk" of God's Torah. (305)

Thus, to bare one's breasts in this context is not a desperate act of a crazed woman but rather a reminder of the word of God, written in the Torah, interpreted by scholars and passed down intergenerationally both through the rabbinic tradition and through the sacred role of families – including mothers – in the Jewish tradition. This, Kosman argues, is therefore not an angry protest but rather a "tempering of the masculine experience by the feminine one," which may "also contain an element of supplication" (2004, 307).

Such stories of mothers baring their breasts in defiance of masculine authority are not unique to the Torah, either. Greek literature, including *The Iliad* by Homer, includes examples of bared breasts to represent pleas for mercy. Kosman quotes from *The Libation Bearers* by Aeschylus, when Clytemnestra pleads with her son to stop his vengeance for the murder of Agamemnon: "Hold, my son! Have pity, child, upon this breast at which full oft, sleeping the while, with toothless gums didst suck the milk that nourished thee" (as cited in Kosman 2004, 308).

If breastfeeding holds such archetypical power as a symbol of divine love and mystical connection, you might think women would have had more authority over the course of history. Or perhaps, men might be a wee bit jealous that women get to experience this heavenly act and they don't. However, the physical act of nursing an infant has more often been framed as animalistic, lending evidence to support women's lower status relative to men. Schiebinger reflects, "The notion that a woman – lacking male perfections of mind and body – resides nearer the beast is an ancient one" (1993, 394). She recounts the Roman myth of Romulus and Remus, who were abandoned and saved by sucking at the nipple of a wolf. In *Historia animalium*, Aristotle also linked humans to animals through the breast, along with menstruation and sperm. A similar pattern is found in early Jewish texts, Schiebinger notes, which refer to menstruation and childbirth as "curses, rendering them unclean, undesirable, and beastlike" (394).

Breastfeeding continued to be used as evidence for women's closer proximity to the animal world, leading to visually ambivalent depictions of the act in ancient Rome, according to ancient historian Claude-Emmanuelle Centlivres Challet (2017). Though breastfeeding was essential to human survival, starting at least with Greek physician Soranus of Ephesus in the first or second century, men engaged in strategies to wrest control over breastfeeding away from women as a means to cope with their envy of the power and pleasure they believed breastfeeding brought to women, such as by associating it with animality and suggesting that it made breasts ugly. They also tried to appropriate breastfeeding by creating medical and social rules around it, suggesting that women were too feeble minded to know how to do it properly. For instance, doctors of the day wrongly suggested that colostrum is indigestible and should be discarded. Socially, women were encouraged to use wet nurses to allow them to return to their functions as ladies of the house through further procreation or through socializing to "flaunt the household's social status and wealth." Combining both concerns, Soranus, for instance, argued that "intercourse might spoil a mother's milk, diminish its flow, or suppress it completely[, which] might have prompted decisions to delegate breastfeeding" (Challet 2017, 376). However, he also offered mixed advice as to the use of wet nurses, offering reasons to use them but also stating that "maternal milk is the best milk and that it should only be replaced with another woman's milk if the mother is unable to breastfeed" (377). Thus, though breastfeeding was associated with the Divine, breastfeeding was to be left to the poor and peasant class, not to the "ladies."

It seems obvious in a way that breastfeeding would be the metaphorical referent for milk and honey: there are no humans who have ever lived without some mother's milk and honey, but plenty have lived at arm's length from bees or goats. I do appreciate that there is something divinely comforting about breasts. Is there anything more soothing than a big hug from a generously endowed older woman? And when they were little my kids did seem to prefer resting their heads on my soft bosom over their father's bony sternum. Or, as the British indie rock band Cornershop (1997) sing in their hit single "Brimful of Asha," "everybody needs a bosom for a pillow." I can see why a suffering people would seek refuge in the image of a comforting breast of an all-loving God. However, as we will see in the next chapter, the metaphorical usage of breasts and breastfeeding became a particularly insidious tool in seizing power from women in the transition to capitalism.

4 Witches' Brews and Breasts

But first let us consider the smallest of these injuries, that of drying up the milk. If it is asked how they can do this, it can be answered that, according to Blessed Albert in his Book on Animals, milk is naturally menstrual in any animal; and, like another flux in women, when it is not stopped by some natural infirmity, it is due to witchcraft that it is stopped. Now the flow of milk is naturally stopped when the animal becomes pregnant; and it is stopped by an accidental infirmity when the animal eats some herb the nature of which is to dry up the milk and make the cow ill. But they can cause this in various ways by witchcraft. For on the more holy nights according to the instructions of the devil and for the greater offence to the Divine Majesty of God, a witch will sit down in a corner of her house with a pail between her legs, stick a knife or some instrument in the wall or a post, and make as if to milk it with her hands. Then she summons her familiar who always works with her in everything and tells him that she wishes to milk a certain cow from a certain house, which is healthy and abounding in milk. And suddenly the devil takes the milk from the udder of that cow, and brings it to where the witch is sitting, as if it were flowing from the knife …

Also, because when witches wish to deprive a cow of milk they are in the habit of begging a little of the milk or butter which comes from that cow, so that they may afterwards by their art bewitch the cow; therefore women should take care, when they are asked by persons suspected of this crime, not to give away the least thing to them.

Heinrich Kramer and James Sprenger, "Here followeth how Witches Injure Cattle in Various Ways," *Malleus Maleficarum*, Part II

As explored in the previous chapter, ancient and early religious symbolism surrounding breasts and breastfeeding have been discursively framed in terms of their divine, or sometimes earthly, nature. However, whatever ways this framing was used to dominate or control the female body was radically accelerated and intensified during the Middle Ages. In her riveting book, *Caliban and the Witch*, Italian feminist theorist Silvia Federici (2014) argues that controlling women's bodies was essential to the transition from the feudal system of the

Middle Ages to the rise of early capitalism. Federici demonstrates that capitalism was made possible only as a result of class struggle and the mass murder and torture of women. Though she draws on Marx's critique of capitalist development as contingent on the creation and suppression of a working class, she identifies an important lacuna in his (and most others') theories for failing to explore the witch hunts as anything other than an historical curiosity. Federici makes a convincing case for the centrality of these events to the functioning of a capitalist social order. I build on her account by examining the use of witches' breasts as a visual ploy used to further advance these economic changes. Not only did this prove useful for early capitalists, but the metaphors developed at the time continue to be a salient means of shaming the non-lactating mother.

Witch Hunts and the Rise of Early Capitalism

Though sites of witch trials are essentially tourist attractions today, Federici (2014) makes clear that there was nothing fun or cute about the witch hunts. Women were shaved, raped, publicly exposed, paraded naked through town, drowned, burned at the stake, put in cages, and otherwise subjected to some of the most sadistic examples of torture known to history. The European witch hunts began in the early fourteenth century and lasted until around 1650, thus from the late Middle Ages to the start of the early modern period. However, the practice of witchcraft, sorcery, or other forms of magical technologies dates back at least to classical Greece and probably earlier. Prior to the witch hunts, witchcraft was a rather non-controversial practice often employed to produce good outcomes or prevent bad ones, throughout many parts of the world. In fact, according to sociologist Nachman Ben-Yehuda, the Old Testament is nearly completely silent on witchcraft, with two exceptions: "the 'Witch of Endor' with whom King Saul consulted before his last battle (1 Sam. 28:9)" and the commandment from Exodus 22:10 that "Thou shalt not suffer a witch to live" (1980, 2). Beyond these two mentions, "however, all stories [in the Bible] concerning witches are neutral in the sense that witches, devils, and demons are never elaborately conceptualized, and the existence of an all-encompassing supernatural, demonic world is never mentioned" (2). Further, Christian authorities did not acknowledge the existence of witches from 900 to 1400 CE, despite a popular belief in them throughout the Middle Ages (Leeson and Russ 2018). Thus, the creation of the witch as "Satan's puppet" was new when it emerged in the fourteenth century along with a new theory of demonology, which enabled "the inquisitors, and other individuals, to persecute legitimately hundreds of thousands of witches" (Ben-Yehuda 1980, 3).

Though smaller witch trials were reported as early as 1245, the movement to hunt witches is seen as growing from the fourteenth and fifteenth centuries and finding its heyday after the 1490s. According to Leeson and Russ, "Sixty per cent were prosecuted between 1560 and 1630, a period known as the 'Great hunt'; more than half within a 300-mile radius of Strasbourg, France" (2018, 2067). Spain, Italy, and Portugal largely avoided witch trials (Leeson and Russ 2018), while Germany, Switzerland, and France had some of the worst (Ben-Yehuda 1980). The movement to persecute witches was encouraged most notably by the publication of the *Malleus Malefi-carum* (*The witch's hammer*) in 1486, quoted at the start of this chapter. This handbook on how to identify and persecute witches was written by two Dominican friars, Heinrich Kramer and James (also Jacob) Sprenger ([1486] 1928), in response to Pope Innocent VIII's issuance of a papal bull recognizing witches and sorcery as real. According to Ben-Yehuda,

> The main feature of the European witch craze was the "Witches' Sabbath," the climax of which was a huge orgy between the devil and witches; at this time new witches were initiated. The ceremony allegedly included denying salvation, kissing the devil's posterior, spitting on the Bible, having promiscuous sexual orgies, feasting on roasted or boiled unbaptized children's flesh and exhumed corpses, mocking the holy sacrament of baptism, cursing the cross, and the like. (1980, 5)

Thus, it was during this time that witchcraft went from a neutral technology to support crop growth and such to an anti-religion that sought to subvert Christianity through mocking and negatively mirroring Christian rituals and symbols (for instance, by kissing the "he-goat's posterior" instead of kissing the cross, or by playing spooky organ music instead of hymns) (6).

Though there are a multitude of explanations for what sparked the witch trials, what is clear is that they were not simply a result of mass panic or a "craze" (Horsley and Horsley 1987, 21) brought on by ignorance or even simple misogyny. Such explanations fail to explain why the witch hunt emerged when and where it did. However, there is rather compelling evidence that the witch hunts were a strategy for taking land and centralizing wealth and power. Although most theorists of capitalism, including Karl Marx, have entirely ignored the relevance of this systematic gynocide, Federici (2014) points out that the historical context of the witch trials coincides with the emergence of early capitalism.

Primitive Capital Accumulation

Marx ([1867] 1977) is a foundational and central thinker within the field of sociology precisely for his otherwise comprehensive theoretical analysis of the emergence and future of capitalism. He theorized that capitalism was only able to emerge when wealth (capital) could be concentrated within the hands of a small elite class, who used power and force to separate workers from the means of production. In order for owners (the bourgeoisie) to expand their wealth, they had to take control of how work would be carried out. They needed to own the factory and have workers labour within it to expand the owners' wealth beyond what any individual could produce alone. As such, force – including physical violence, disenfranchisement, and other control techniques – became the main lever of economic expansion. The witch trials were just one of many tactics that successfully forced peasants off the common land, separated artisans from their shops and guilds, and claimed territorial ownership. The taking of property and debasing of the rights of workers ensured inexpensive and ample labour power to further enrich the owners. This is why we see the reinstitution of "slavery and other forms of coerced labor as the dominant work relation" (Federici 2014, 64) in the first three hundred years of capitalism in the United States and throughout Europe. Throughout Europe, where slavery was less prevalent, owners found alternative means of exploitation by taking lands and then forcing waged labour onto the peasantry. However, these harsh and exploitative working conditions introduced a serious contradiction: how to keep labour costs as low as possible, without abusing workers so much that they became inefficient at the job, quit, or died. As Federici notes,

> This contradiction – which still characterizes capitalist development – exploded most dramatically in the American colonies, where work, disease, and disciplinary punishments destroyed two thirds

of the Native American population in the decades immediately after the Conquest. It was also at the core of the slave trade and the exploitation of slave labor. Millions of Africans died because of the torturous living conditions to which they were subjected during the Middle Passage and on the plantations. (2014, 65–6)

Not only were early capitalists testing the limits of exploitation and abuse of workers, but former peasants were also being starved by the loss of common lands. Beginning in the twelfth century in England, and then rapidly spreading from roughly 1450 to 1640 (notably, the exact same time as the bulk of the witch hunts), the "enclosure movement" involved the privatization of lands by landed nobility in order to concentrate their wealth and power. These previously commonly used areas – places where the peasantry could farm, fish, or hunt for food, in order to maintain at least a minimal subsistence life – were now being "enclosed," or closed off to the public. Along with wildly fluctuating prices of goods without commensurate increases in wages, the enclosure movement meant that many of the peasantry began to go hungry owing to repeated famines throughout Europe (Federici 2014; Fischer 1996). The starvation was so dire that multitudes of mothers and children took to the streets begging for food or stealing what they could. Additionally, because women were most likely to be the ones in charge of feeding their children, and younger mothers were busy with said children, grandmothers tended to be the ones to initiate and lead peasant food revolts. Federici describes how "the main weapons available to the poor in their struggle for survival were their own famished bodies, as in times of famine hordes of vagabonds and beggars surrounded the better off, half-dead of hunger and disease, grabbing their arms, exposing their wounds to them, and forcing them to live in a state of constant fear at the prospect of both contamination and revolt" (2014, 81).

As a means to control the starving masses and avoid revolt, the state began to enact various forms of public assistance in the early sixteenth century. Although marking "the first recognition of the unsustainability of a capitalist system ruling exclusively by means of hunger and terror," public assistance programs also let the owners and elite class off the hook by shifting "ownership" of workers from employers to the state, "enabling employers to relinquish any responsibility for the reproduction of workers" (Federici 2014, 84). By "reproduction," Federici means the daily reproductive needs, like feeding, housing, or other caring responsibilities of workers;

many early factories had required workers to live on-site in dormitories, where they would be fed but their every hour could be controlled.

During this period, social science emerged as the state began to take an interest in demographic data, allowing for the tracking of population-level trends through censuses and the collection of data on birth, marriage, or death rates. As government spending increased to address the social problems that came with capitalist development, heated debates proliferated around the world regarding who would qualify as the deserving poor, who should be provided with social supports, and who would be deemed an able-bodied worker. One solution was the creation of workhouses to justify welfare payments from the state. As the state dabbled in how best to create a welfare state, workers, including children and the elderly, "became the experimental subjects for a variety of work-schemes" (Federici 2014, 85), and we begin to see the criminalizing of an expanding proletariat.

The European capitalist quest for cheap labour continued to prove challenging owing to worker resistance and death, brought on not only by famine but also by the arrival of the Black Death in the mid-1300s. Capitalist hopes for access to a new mass of exploitable labour after Columbus' "discovery" of the New World were further dashed with the near total decimation of Indigenous peoples throughout North and South America within one hundred years. Federici discusses the impact of this demographic and economic crisis:

> It is my contention that it was the population crisis of the 16th and 17th centuries ... that turned reproduction and population growth into state matters, as well as primary objects of intellectual discourse. I further argue that the intensification of the persecution of "witches," and the new disciplinary methods that the state adopted in this period to regulate procreation and break women's control over reproduction, are also to be traced to this crisis. (2014, 86)

While acknowledging that there were likely many fears that drove the witch hunts, Federici makes the rather compelling claim that "it cannot be a pure coincidence, however, that at the very moment when population was declining, and an ideology was forming that stressed the centrality of labor in economic life, severe penalties were introduced in the legal codes of Europe to punish women guilty of reproductive crimes" (2014,

87). Specifically, more women "were executed for infanticide in 16th and 17th-century Europe than for any other crime except for witchcraft, a charge that also centered on the killing of children and other violations of reproductive norms." During this time, childbirth, long under the purview of midwives, began to be taken over by male doctors. The new role of midwives became policing women under the supervision of doctors. In France and Germany, the state used midwives to spy on new mothers and to "examine suspected local women for any signs of lactation when foundlings were discovered on the Church's steps." As Federici writes, "While in the Middle Ages women had been able to use various forms of contraceptives, and had exercised undisputed control over the birthing process, from now on their wombs became public territory, controlled by men and the state, and procreation was directly placed at the service of capitalist accumulation" (89).

In this way, Federici argues that under capitalism, women's bodies came to be understood as valuable assets in expanding the availability of labour in both Europe and early American colonial plantations. Though there were significant differences, in that African slave mothers were openly delivered for rape and their children taken away and sold on the auction block (Roberts [1997] 2014), in both contexts women could be raped with impunity and their bodies "turned into an instrument for the reproduction of labor and the expansion of the work-force, treated as natural breeding-machines, functioning according to rhythms outside of women's control" (Federici 2014, 91).

One particularly important mechanism for obtaining women's "free" labour in reproducing workers was the devaluation of women's paid work and creation of a cultural value of marriage as "women's true career." A particularly salient route through which women's labour could be devalued was the criminalization of sex work. With the elimination of the commons and the exodus of women from rural to urban areas, prostitution became "the main form of subsistence for a large female population." Not for long, however; as Federici writes,

Whereas in the late Middle Ages it had been officially accepted as a necessary evil, and prostitutes had benefited from the high wage regime, in the 16th century, the situation was reversed. In a climate of intense misogyny, characterized by the advance of the Protestant Reformation and witch-hunting, prostitution was first subjected to new restrictions and then criminalized. Everywhere, between

1530–1560, town brothels were closed and prostitutes, especially
street-walkers, were subjected to severe penalties: banishment,
flogging, and other cruel forms of chastisement ... Meanwhile, in
16th-century France, the raping of a prostitute ceased to be a crime.
(2014, 94)

Not only was a significant means of survival taken away from large
numbers of women, but women also began to be forced out of guilds by
craftsmen angry at the capitalist class who had begun paying women lower
wages. As detailed by Federici (2014), "Whether in Italy, France, or Germany, journeymen petitioned the authorities not to allow women to com-
pete with them, banned them from their ranks, went on strike when the
ban was not observed, and even refused to work with men who worked
with women." This was then further reinforced by messages in popular
culture depicting these European women who worked outside the home
as "sexually aggressive shrews" (96). And all of this with the full cooperation of authorities. As Federici argues,

It was from this alliance between the crafts and the urban authorities, along with the continuing privatization of land, that a new
sexual division of labor or, better, a new "sexual contract," in Carol
Pateman's words (1988), was forged, defining women in terms –
mothers, wives, daughters, widows – that hid their status as workers,
while giving men free access to women's bodies, their labor, and the
bodies and labor of their children ... This was for women a historic
defeat ... For in pre-capitalist Europe women's subordination to men
had been tempered by the fact that they had access to the commons
and other communal assets, while in the new capitalist regime
women themselves became the commons. (97)

Vain and Wicked Women

As the state began to assert control over women's bodies, popular rhetoric
surrounding women grew increasingly virulent, as noted by Federici:

Women were accused of being unreasonable, vain, wild, wasteful.
Especially blamed was the female tongue, seen as an instrument of
insubordination. But the main female villain was the disobedient
wife, who, together with the "scold," the "witch," and the "whore"

was the favorite target of dramatists, popular writers, and moralists. In this sense, Shakespeare's *The Taming of the Shrew* (1593) was the manifesto of the age. (2014, 100–1)

Nothing was so successful at the taming of women than the great witch hunt. As the general public was increasingly primed to see women, especially older women, as selfish, crazy, and wicked old crones, framing them as literal witches was a short leap. This was further facilitated by Biblical depictions of Eve, easily tempted by the evil serpent at the expense of an extended stay in Eden, coupled with a pre-existing and widely shared cultural belief in mysticism and/or superstitions. At this time, women were more likely than men to be called upon to recite incantations and perform rituals in the hopes of improving crop yields, controlling unruly livestock, or ensuring the safe delivery of a baby (Betea 2015).

In this way, witch hunts provided a powerful means by which to disable the power of an increasingly discontented working class. Federici (2014) cites three conditions that correlated with witch trials during this period: rising food prices (first documented by Kamen [1972]), the taking of previously common land for private ownership (the enclosure movement), and times of peasant revolt triggered by the first two conditions. Considering that women were endowed with the responsibility for feeding their children, it makes sense that rising food prices coupled with limited access to the commons would lead peasant women to risk their lives to "protect their children from starvation" (Federici 2014, 174). As Federici writes, "the persecution of witches grew on this terrain. It was a class war carried out by other means" (176). In other words, suppression of women through torture and genocide was a means of suppressing peasant/worker insurrection.

While actual women were fighting the powerful to save their starving children, cultural depictions of evil witches – childless old crones feeding at midnight Sabbaths on the bodies of dead babies – began to circulate popularly. According to Patricia Simons,

Central to many treatises, accusations, and confessions was the secret gathering or witches' Sabbath, often in a remote location, at which loyalty was pledged to the devil ... Common too were stories of night flight, infanticide, and cannibalism, the use of potions, the manipulation of impotence or fertility or desire, sexual intercourse with *incubi* or *succubi*, the rousing of storms, the killing of animals, or instruction in magic, all of which appear in varying degrees in classical accounts as well, though in more scattered passages and primarily in literary rather than historical contexts. (2015, 265)

In addition to being non-procreative and actively infanticidal, these depictions transgress the boundaries established by capitalism around the workday. Federici cites the conclusions of Italian philosopher Luciano Parinetto (1998), who identifies numerous ways in which the characteristics demonized in witches are those that threaten the development of capitalist discipline: "Parinetto points out that the nocturnal dimension of the Sabbat was a violation of the contemporary capitalist regularization of work-time, and a challenge to private property and sexual orthodoxy, as the night shadows blurred the distinctions between the sexes and between 'mine and thine'" (Federici 2014, 177).

Whereas in Europe men were spared from accusations of witchcraft, enslaved Black men in the United States were terrorized by accusations of participating in witchcraft while, unlike European White women, explicitly treated as property. The anti-miscegenation laws of the 1660s, for instance, drew on tropes of the witch and the Black devil, to frame Black men as bogeymen whom White women should fear. Most colonizers in North and South America worked to enforce a sexual hierarchy wherein men would dominate women and children, except for enslaved Africans; only among this group did men and women face a kind of equal opportunity for horrifying brutality (Federici 2014).

Colonial rule and exploitation for European capitalist profit was also not limited to the US slave system. The Spanish colonists tried to "divide and rule" by creating new racial hierarchies between White, Indigenous, and mixed race (*mestizo*) peoples, via laws around property rights and inheritance and restrictions on intermarriage. The Jesuits in seventeenth-century New France, now Canada, worked to "Christianize" the Naskapi Indigenous peoples by teaching men to control their wives and beat their children, in part by defining disobedient wives as "creatures of the devil." Federici further suggests that the important differences in the treatment of enslaved Black men versus Indigenous men was in the desired usage of the men's bodies by Europeans:

The Montagnais-Naskapi men owed their training in male supremacy to the fact that the French wanted to instill in them the "instinct" for private property, to induce them to become reliable partners in the fur trade. Very different was the situation on the plantations, where the sexual division of labor was immediately dictated by the planters' requirements for labor-power, and by the price of commodities produced by the slaves on the international market. (2014, 111)

In both the American colonies and in Europe, an explicit aim of the witch hunts was to control women's reproductive capacity; the most common crime witches were accused of were infanticide and preventing conception. Further, witches were often described as having powers to emasculate men, by stealing their penises or at least make them impotent. In the *Malleus Maleficarum*, an entire chapter is devoted to the question of "Whether Witches may work some Prestidigatory Illusion so that the Male Organ appears to be entirely removed and separate from the Body" (Kramer and Sprenger [1486] 1928, Part 1, Question IX). Perhaps this is why, aside from individual male relatives, only one male organization – a group of fishermen in the Basque region – was recorded to have come to the aid of women accused of witchcraft. Most other men took it upon themselves to serve as "witch hunters," or to use a witch hunt as an opportunity "to free themselves of unwanted wives and lovers, or to blunt the revenge of women they had raped or seduced" (Federici 2014, 189). European men could be persecuted for aiding and abetting their purported witch family members, "but there is no doubt that years of propaganda and terror sowed among men the seeds of a deep psychological alienation from women, that broke class solidarity and undermined their own collective power" (189).

Thus, the witch hunts were not only effective at claiming territory and dividing and conquering the proletariat; they were also notable for managing to claim and control the bodies of White, Black, Indigenous, and other colonized women, as well as enslaved Black men. As Federici notes,

Just as the Enclosures expropriated the peasantry from the communal land, so the witch-hunt expropriated women from their bodies, which were thus "liberated" from any impediment preventing them to function as machines for the production of labor. For the threat of the stake erected more formidable barriers around women's bodies than were ever erected by the fencing off of the commons. (184, her italics)

Witches' Breasts

Confirmation that a woman was a witch often relied on identifying physical characteristics of a woman's body that were said to prove exactly that. Breasts were among the most symbolically powerful of them. Fascinatingly, one of the greatest consistencies in the depictions of evil witches is the shrivelled breasts of an old crone, which sharply contrast to images of the divine nursing mother portrayed with full and luscious breasts, as discussed in the previous chapter and as shown in Albrecht Dürer's 1510–11 *The Life of the Virgin* (figure 4.1). To provide another example, as depicted in Zwolle's etching below (figure 4.2), twelfth-century Saint Bernard of Clairvaux was said to have been visited by Mary, who then "expressed some of her breast milk into his lips, thus enabling him to spread the word of Christ with such beauty and conviction that all who heard were unable to resist" (Kissin 1991, 454).

In contrast to this idealized, good breast, witches were depicted with ugly, drooping, and flaccid breasts, clearly devoid of any healing powers. In describing the etching *Four Witches* (1515), likely by Hans Frank of Basel (figure 4.3), Charles Zika writes, "The physical destruction wrought by witchcraft is graphically embodied in the emaciated figure of the standing witch with distended breasts and a child tied to her back by her hair ... She is clearly menopausal, a representation of anti-nurture, bearing what is presumably a dead child" (2007, 84).

German artists Albrecht Dürer (1471–1528) and Hans Baldung Grien (circa 1484–1545) were arguably the two artists most devoted to depicting witches with drooping breasts, which they made even droopier over the course of their careers. Dürer first introduced the young naked witch with his engraving *Four Witches* in 1497 (figure 4.4), followed three years later by *Witch Riding Backward on a Goat* (figure 4.5). Noticeably, the earlier piece portrays bodies with relatively young-looking breasts, albeit not the most abundant, especially compared with the goat-riding hag's breasts.

Given that Baldung worked under Dürer from about 1503 to 1507 (Sullivan 2000), the influence the latter had on the former should be unsurprising. Thus, in Baldung's *The Witches* (figure 4.6) from 1510, we see a similar depiction of younger and more pert breasts contrasting with the older drooping breasts of the scariest-looking witch. In Baldung's *Bewitched Groom*, circa 1544 (figure 4.7), we see a perhaps satirical image of a witch

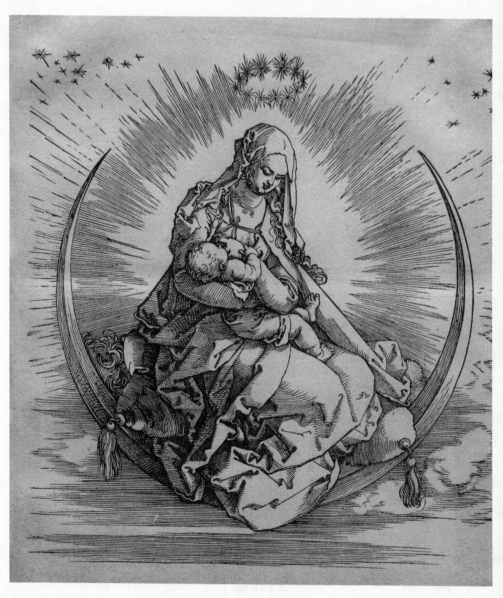

4.1 *The Life of the Virgin*, by Albrecht Dürer, circa 1510–11.

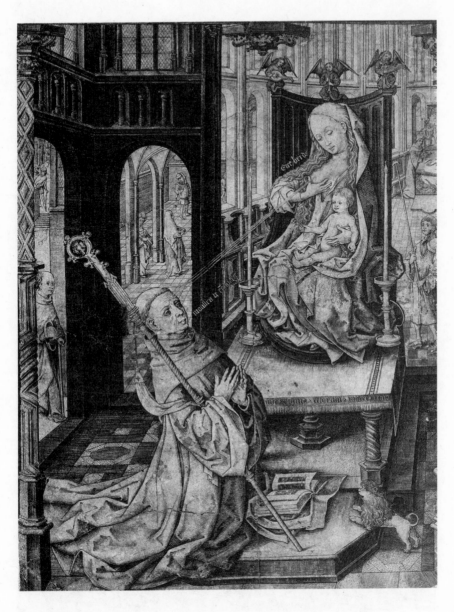

4.2 *The Lactation of Saint Bernard of Clairvaux*, by Master I.A.M. of Zwolle, circa 1480–85.

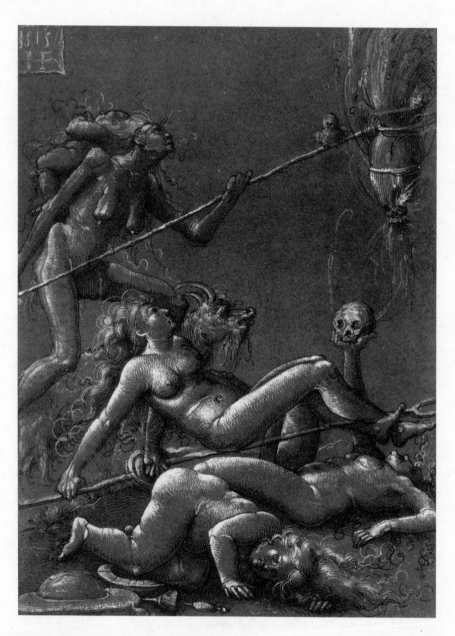

4.3 *Four Witches*, likely by Hans Ulrich Franck of Basel, 1515.

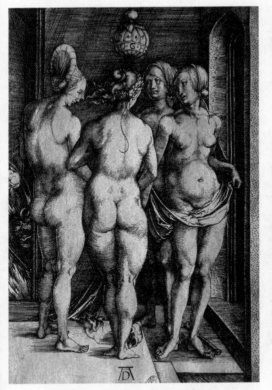
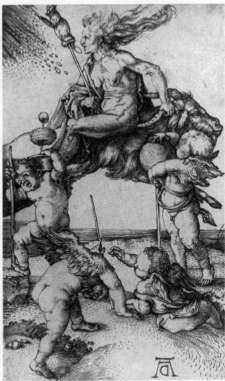

4.4 *The Four Witches,* by Albrecht Dürer, 1497.

4.5 *Witch Riding Backward on a Goat Accompanied by Four Putti,* by Albrecht Dürer, circa 1505.

who has subdued a man to the floor (notably with his codpiece centred in the image), with an old witch waving a broom or torch with her breasts bared outside of her clothing, which Patricia Emison suggests is used "to parody the Triumph of Women *topos*" (1999, 625).

Interestingly, Dürer's goat-riding witch is said to have been inspired by Andrea Mantegna's portrayal of the ancient goddess Envy in his earlier engraving, *Battle of the Sea Gods* (circa 1475–88) (figure 4.8), which also shows a monstrous emaciated woman with stretched out, sagging, phallic breasts. In Envy's hand hangs a sign with the word "Invidia," referencing the ancient Roman poet Ovid's Invidia, a woman with an evil eye who casts envy in the hearts of those who dare look into it (Simons 2015).

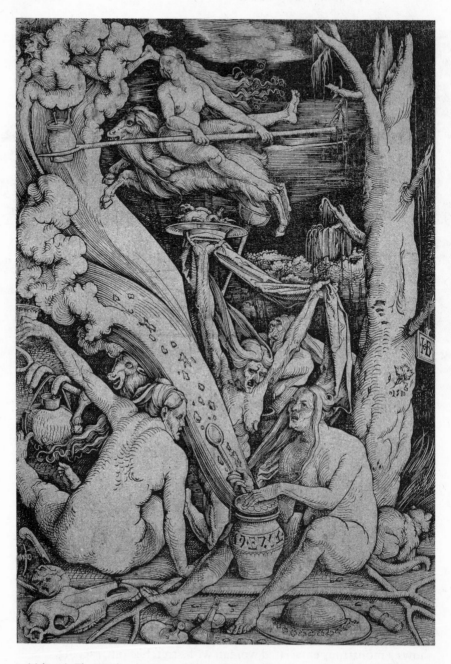

4.6 (above) *The Witches*, by Hans Baldung Grien, 1510.

4.7 (facing) *The Bewitched Groom*, by Hans Baldung Grien, 1544–45.

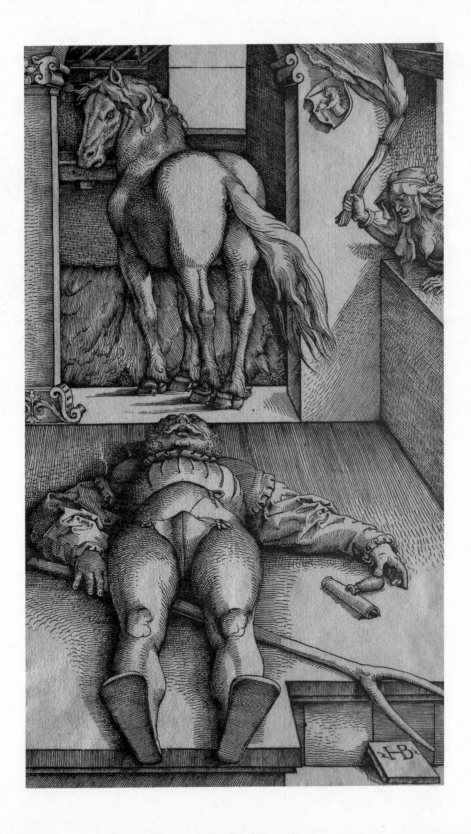

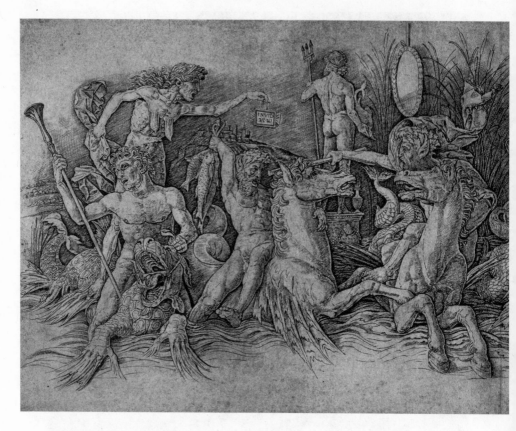

4.8 *Battle of the Sea Gods*, left portion, by Andrea Mantegna, circa 1485–88.

The witches of Dürer, Baldung, and Mantegna contain many similarities to witches depicted by earlier poets and artists, with one significant innovation: the depiction of their breasts. The artists' usage of drooping, sagging breasts was a new contribution not found in classical art or rhetoric. According to Simons, wizened breasts

rarely appear in classical or medieval culture, and when they do, they are not associated with witches; and only in the unusual case of a few obscure figurines, unknown during the Renaissance, is Envy perhaps shown thus. Rather, the exaggeratedly empty breasts signify ugliness, extreme old age, or the allegorical figure of Fury. The combination of witch with Envy and with drooping breasts takes place over the course of the sixteenth century, bringing together misogyny and allegory, blending ancient and medieval strands. By the

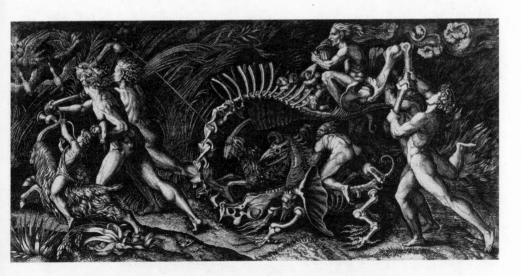

4.9 *Lo Stregozzo* (*The Carcass*), likely by Agostino Veneziano, circa 1515–25.

late fifteenth century, and even more widely by the 1530s, the aged
woman with shrunken breasts had become the stock figure of Envy,
and by the 1580s this visual rhetoric was perhaps a sign of the witch.
The thin, ugly old woman, in other words, is not always a witch.
The promiscuous, ugly, and often old woman is a staple of ancient
Roman invective, frequently accused of having a loose vagina (from
overuse) and overlarge breasts. (2015, 291)

This trend of the drooping breast to signal a witch was also seen in other
parts of Europe and around the world. For instance, the Italian engraving
Lo Stregozzo (*The Carcass*) from 1515–25 (figure 4.9), likely made by Agostino Veneziano, was also said to be influenced by both Dürer's *Witch Riding
Backward on a Goat* (1500) and Mantegna's *Battle of the Sea Gods* (1475–88)
and depicts a witch with significantly sagging breasts.

Rangda, the Indonesian Witch

The tell-tale drooping breast characterizes another culturally iconic witch
during this era, though halfway around the world in Indonesia: Rangda,
a hideous anti-maternal widow witch, her name itself meaning "widow"
(Hannigan 2015). Anthropologist Clifford Geertz describes her portrayal in
live performances in the Indonesian province of Bali:

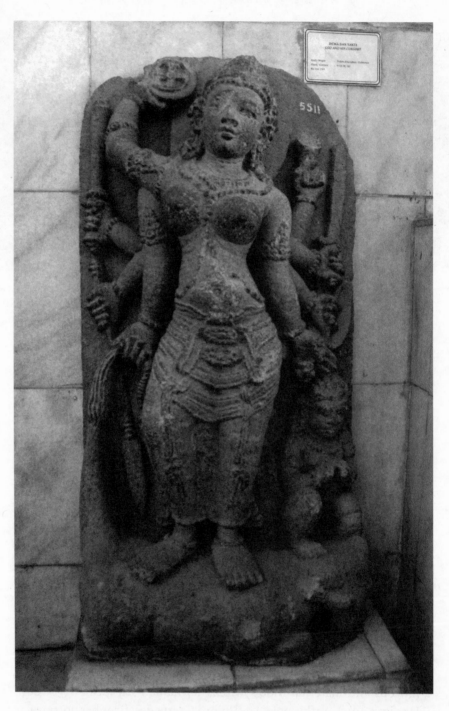

4.10 Relief of the Hindu goddess Durga, circa 700s–800s.

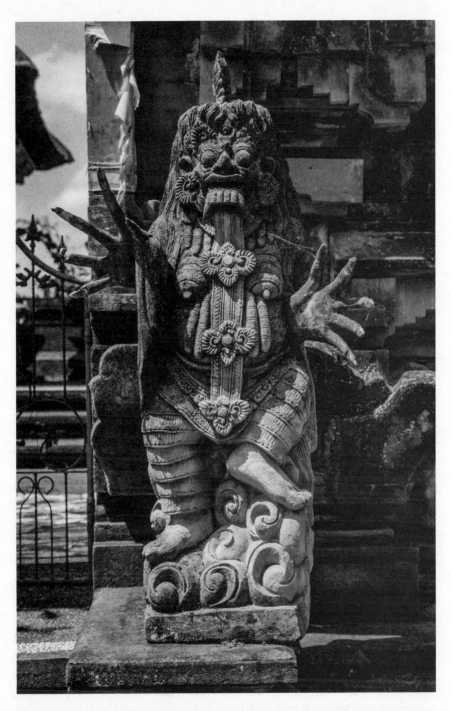

4.11 Stone statue of Rangda, Indonesia.

Rangda, danced by a single male, is a hideous figure. Her eyes bulge from her forehead like swollen boils. Her teeth become tusks curving up over her cheeks and fangs protruding down her chin. Her yellowed hair falls down around her in a matted tangle. Her breasts are dry and pendulous dugs edged with hair, between which hang, like so many sausages, strings of colored entrails. (1973, 114)

The origins and meaning of Rangda are unclear, according to Geertz, but one explanation suggests that "Rangda is an incarnation of Durga, Siva's malignant consort" (1973, 117), who is sometimes depicted as a frightening goddess capable of bringing or preventing death. Francine Brinkgreve notes that "visual images of Durga in, for example, reliefs, sculptures, and (magic) drawings, often depict the goddess in the same monstrous form as Rangda" (1997, 242). The physical differences between the Hindu goddess Durga and the Balinese witch Rangda are clear in their artistic representations, as the goddess Durga "is usually depicted as a beautiful eight-armed woman standing on top of a buffalo" (243). Sarah Weiss adds that "the goddess Durga is depicted with a beatific and voluptuous demeanour on Hindu temples in the region, her face is calm and her body relaxed and sensual" (2017, 53). Notably, the Hindu goddess Durga is depicted with pert breasts, whereas Rangda always has drooping, sagging breasts.

The transformation of the Balinese goddess Durga into Rangda seems to have coincided with the end of the Majapahit period in Indonesia, sometime between the late fourteenth and early sixteenth centuries (S. Weiss 2017). The Catholic Portuguese began their Christian mission and economic exploration and crusades in this same period, starting in 1511. I have no smoking gun to prove that Portuguese (or later Dutch) explorers transformed Durga into Rangda, but there are several interesting dots that we can connect. For one, the Portuguese period in Indonesia began less than twenty-five years after the publication of the *Malleus Maleficarum* in Germany. Further, Portugal sent Roman Catholic explorers and missionaries such as Francis Xavier to Indonesia in the early sixteenth century. And, Francis Xavier was said to have written King João III of Portugal in 1546 to try to persuade him to spread the Inquisition to Goa, India – the South Asian centre of Portuguese colonialism from where many of the Indonesian explorers began their crusades (Hannigan 2015). This is why, according to Tim Hannigan, the Portuguese can be seen as the "founding fathers of European colonialism in Southeast Asia ... [casting] a brittle arc of Catholicism through the easternmost islands" (2015, 81).

By 1602 the Dutch East India Company had been awarded a monopoly on trade by the Dutch Parliament, allowing the Dutch in 1619 to conquer an area they named Batavia, now called Jakarta. While I cannot offer definitive proof that either Dürer or Baldung or the Portuguese or Dutch explorers were a direct cause, the transformation of a goddess of destruction, to whom local people prayed, into a terrifying baby-eating witch, with drooping breasts similar to those depicted on witches in the colonizing country, does not seem coincidental.

Hunger and the Empty Breast

Further evidence to support Federici's (2014) contention that capitalist development required the disciplining of women's bodies, and that this is what explains the witch hunts in history, is to be found in Sullivan's (2000) defence of Dürer and Baldung. In an effort to show that Baldung's work was influenced more by the German humanists than by the *Malleus Maleficarum* or any other guide to demonology, Sullivan suggests that there "is wit and humor in Baldung's drawings of witches, qualities not characteristic of the witchcraft manuals and folklore stories although these have remained the focus of scholarly attention. Koerner remarks the 'comic tone' of Baldung's witches" (363). Thus, she suggests that theirs are works of satire and should not be viewed as having contributed to or supportive of the witch hunts. To further her point, she details what Baldung's life was like:

> Baldung's innovations are consistent with the humanist climate in which he lived, worked, and found patrons. Even a brief survey of his art, early training, and the audience available to him make this humanist orientation apparent. Baldung was born around 1485 and raised in academic and intellectual circles with his family occupying an important place in Strasbourg society ...
> As a young man Baldung worked with Dürer at Nuremberg from around 1503 to 1507, during a period when the "Poets" and humanist sodalities were active in the city, and Dürer had just broken new ground with his witch prints. These were among the first of Dürer's works to which the younger artist was exposed, a time when he might be especially susceptible to the older artist's influence, and Dürer remained a central point of reference for Baldung, an interest that was reciprocated as Dürer gave away prints by "Hans Grien"

during his visit to the Low Countries in 1520–1521 and when Dürer died in 1528 it was thought appropriate to send Baldung a lock of his hair.

After leaving Dürer's workshop and returning to Strasbourg Baldung prospered, purchasing annuities and speculating in real estate, and he remained an establishment figure throughout his lifetime. By 1527 at the latest, and for the next twenty years, he and his wife had a home in the Brandgasse with neighbors who were "the cream of Strasbourg society," nobility, patricians, and wealthy merchants. Working for "all sectors of the urban and rural ruling classes" in this period of social upheaval, Baldung stood "on the side of property, respectability and order," and his prominent role in the guild, *Zur Steltz*, and election as their representative to the privy council in 1545, as well as various economic documents, attest to his wealth, reputation, and prominence. (Sullivan 2000, 364–6)

This rather extended quote makes clear that both Baldung and Dürer ran in bourgeois elite social circles. Given Federici's (2014) analysis of the purpose of the witch hunts, the two men's lives seem less to exonerate their art as culpable for "creating a climate that could culminate in a tragedy of immense proportions" (Sullivan 2000, 395) than to further solidify the notion that their work was indeed terrible, but in no way ironic.

I would offer further evidence for this by considering why these bourgeois artists might have seen it relevant to transform the classical full breast of the ancient witch into the flaccid, wrinkled bladders of the early modern witch. This change is particularly curious considering that witches were typically associated with sexual promiscuity, said to entice men to engage in illicit activities at night-time orgies. Why not depict the witches with sexually alluring, pert breasts, as the artists had done in other images of non-witches? Perhaps one could counter that the ugly breasts are simply a metaphor for ugliness. We do see in Baldung's *The Witches* (figure 4.6) a depiction of an ugly old crone next to the more sexually alluring, voluptuous younger witches, so maybe. However, there were earlier witches that were plenty ugly without showing bare breasts. Rather, I suggest that the sagging breast was an important scapegoat for the rising food insecurity caused by the transition to capitalism.

We can see the transition in the visual iconography of witches over time in the *De lamiis et pythonicis mulieribus*, a 1489 treatise on witchcraft by

Ulrich Molitor published in the German town of Strasbourg, a hub of interest in witchcraft and home of Hans Baldung Grien (Kwan 2012). There was such interest that the book was printed in at least thirty-nine editions, outnumbering the better known *Malleus Maleficarum*, though this may be partly due to its translation into German (whereas the *Malleus* was printed only in Latin at the time). Though the images did not always match the text, according to Natalie Kwan (2012), the numerous woodcut engravings depicting witchcraft in the *De lamiis* not only helped to "cement the image of the witch" in the minds of the readers but also help us to see how witch iconography changed over time. Kwan notes that prior to the mid-sixteenth century, there was no one coherent image of the witch; thus, woodcuts would include images of male witches and often featured witches transforming into animals. However, by 1544 we see a consistent illustration of naked witches with drooping breasts near cauldrons, feasting during their evening Sabbaths. Kwan describes the 1544 edition of the *De lamiis*, printed by Jakob Cammerlander:

> Unlike the flat-chested women of the earlier De lamiis illustrations, Cammerlander's witch is voluptuous; her sexuality and fertility is linked to her supernatural power. The tension between the witch as temptress and hag is reflected by the witch on the right with her sagging breasts. Instead of the fecund and nurturing woman, the witch embodied the dangers of both the sexually active and post-menopausal woman: envious, lustful and insatiable, she fed on others' fertility and sucked them dry. The witch symbolized the inversion of established moral and sexual order. (510)

Like Kwan, Simons also links the iconography of breasts to fertility, noting that "although breastmilk was not literally reproductive, it was allegorized as a sign of abundance; and in medical discourse, a link was drawn between the uterus and the breast" (2015, 6). However, I would suggest another possible, perhaps more literal, reading of the breast, not as sexual but as a food source – and thus the witch's empty breast to be associated more with food insecurity than sexual deviance, or perhaps with both.

This theory seems supported by Federici's (2014) argument that the witch hunt was a means to divide the proletariat, by destroying the power of grandmother-led rebellions against the widespread starvation resulting from the expanding enclosure movement and rising food prices.

Additionally, Kwan (2012) notes that whereas early imagery of witches was more variable, over hundreds of years the stereotype of a witch changed, in line with Baldung and Dürer's illustrations in the early 1500s of the Sabbath feast. She notes that as time went on, "witchcraft became associated with the New World and cannibalism. Witches were depicted as cruel, old and infertile" (511). Thus, in images of witches' cauldrons, goats, and animal carcasses such as the Italian *Lo Stregozzo* (*The Carcass*) (see fig 4.9) we can see the visual depiction of evil old women controlling and spoiling food supply. Prior to the early modern era,

> early tales of witch gatherings describe an abundance of food and sexual pleasure, partly derived from late antique accusations of promiscuity and cannibalism against the meetings of early Christians, accentuated by folkloric traditions and stories, probably heightened in the case of so-called confessions by the utopian dreams of the poor ... the widespread imagining of idyllic yet sinister banquets was appealing, and permeated high art as much as "popular" fantasy. (Simons 2015, 275)

The fantasy of food must have been immense in a context where starvation was so widespread that "the starving poor, driven to desperation by rising food prices, gathered before the granary in such numbers that some were crushed and others suffocated," as occurred on 19 February 1497 in Florence (Fischer 1996, 68). Following a century and a half of price inflation and resulting starvation, Fischer notes, by the early to mid-sixteenth century, "people sought explanations. Many looked for someone to blame" (1996, 75). I would imagine that people were seeking a scapegoat as soon as they had begun storming the granaries. What better character to blame than the wicked witch?

Given that Dürer and Hans Baldung Grien, like any artist of their day, would have been reliant on the patronage of the well-to-do for their ability to succeed as artists and moved in circles of political and bourgeois elites (Sullivan 2000), we can begin to see reasons for why they would have begun to transform the witch's breast into the crone's drooping udder. In contrast to then recent images of the loving and maternal breast of the Virgin Mary, the witch images associate the breast with diabolical evil. Given the Biblical image of a land of milk and honey in which only mothers can save us from the savagery of life, what could possibly be more terrifying to our most innocent, inner selves than the image of an empty, deflated breast with nothing to offer. Even worse, these anti-mothers parade around naked, baby bones littered around cauldrons of "boiling and frothing white with the swelling foam," as Simons quotes from Ovid's depiction of Medea, "the woman who infamously killed her children" (2015, 284). There is also extensive mythology regarding witches stealing milk from cattle (see, for example, the excerpt from the *Malleus Maleficarum* at the top of this chapter) and other tales of milk-suckling snakes, as witches and devils were also sometimes depicted with snakes (think most obviously of the story of Adam and Eve, which may also be related) (Betea 2015; Ermacora 2017).

Thus, I argue that these "dugs of a crone" have an important role to play not simply in allegorizing the sexual deviance of devil-driven witches but also by offering a salient symbol for starvation. By associating the fear of starvation with women, ruling elites were able to displace blame for social problems away from capitalist accumulation. Further, given the timing, Sullivan (2000) is likely correct that Baldung and Dürer may not have had any direct impact on the witch trials themselves; however, they perhaps fanned the flames for others to express more explicit messages about killing witches.

Not only was this metaphor important for the witch hunts of the pre-modern era, but the psychological priming function of the wizened witch's breast still works today. While actual witch hunts are a rare, though not extinct (Campbell 2019), occurrence around the world, these days we continue to see contrasts made between the good mother with a nursing breast and the bad mother with empty breasts. For example, a basic Google Images search comes up with a seemingly endless supply of happy, breast-feeding mothers, and nowhere is this imagery more prevalent than on breastfeeding promotion websites. At the same time, formula is portrayed literally as a baby killer, such as in the publication of that name (Muller 1974) put out by the British organization War on Want (figure 4.12). In a more recent meme that was making the rounds of the internet, created by a young student blogger, based on no identifiable evidence formula-fed babies were said to be 26.5 per cent more likely to die in the first year than breastfed babies (figure 4.13).

As will be shown in future chapters, such claims are based on very thin scientific evidence, despite volumes of studies suggested to "prove" the benefits of breast milk over formula. I would suggest that part of what has made the anti-formula stance so successful among advocates over the

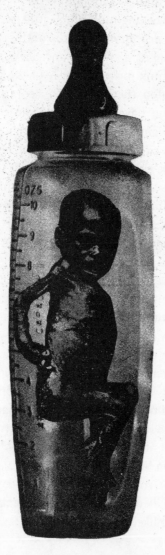

A War on Want investigation into the promotion and sale of powdered baby milks in the Third World

The baby killer

35p

4.12 Cover of "The Baby Killer," 1974.

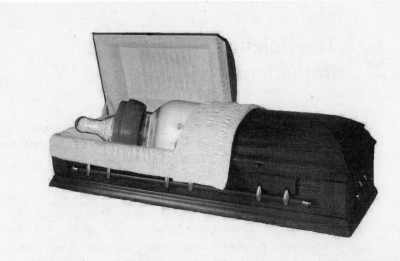

Formula fed babies are 26.5% more likely to die in the first year of life.

Breast is best. The World Health Organization Recommends exclusive breastfeeding
for the first 6 months of life and partial breastfeeding for at least 2 years.

4.13 Internet meme on formula feeding, spreading false information, circa 2014.

past thirty years has less to do with the scientific evidence than with the ability to draw on tropes of the evil witch who is out to kill children. As most breastfeeding advocates suggest, without breastfeeding, babies will die, society will not work, and children will be unruly. As such, women who do not breastfeed threaten moral order with the use of a devilish formula developed to earn money to the detriment of innocent babies. Somewhat ironically, whereas the earlier witches were led by the devil, these modern formula-feeding witches are lured by evil corporations. Just as was done in the Middle Ages, child starvation and death are not attributed to problems in a flawed social or economic structure, but rather to maternal malice, ignorance, or vanity. When infant formula milk is defined as a baby killer or murder weapon (e.g., C. Williams [1939] 1986), mothers who feed their infants formula become baby killers, like the evil witches surrounded by infant carcasses as they stir their pots of white frothing potions.

5 The Science and Nature of Breastfeeding

That the right to breastfeed is even being discussed or challenged, is strange, and even aberrant. It is a challenge to nature, to natural law and natural practice, and to our ecology and environment. Breastfeeding is a natural or God-given (however we may regard nature or god) act. All mammals nearly always feed their young in this way, unless humans prevent them from doing so. All *Mammalian* mothers enjoy this natural practice. All mammals, humans and animals, have the organs and the hormones, the anatomy and physiology, to allow them to nurture their young in this way. That huge numbers of human infants do not get breastfed, and that mothers are influenced not to breastfeed their newborn babies is a distortion of nature. Do not human beings have a right to walk and to run; to laugh and to cry; to breathe the fresh air; and to do a thousand other things using the organs, and body parts, the anatomy and physiology that nature bestowed on them? Females are endowed with breasts, organs designed to produce colostrum and then milk after the birth of a baby, and in a form to allow the infant to feed directly from the mother.

Michael Latham, "Breastfeeding – a Human Rights Issue?"

The violent roots of early modern capitalism underwent a shift beginning in the sixteenth century with the start of a scientific revolution that was exponentially accelerated in the seventeenth century. With the birth of modern science, natural laws and scientific reason crowded out magical thinking and religious ideology, though the latter was by no means displaced in its entirety by the former. Within this new context, no longer could patriarchal and economic power structures rely solely on religious appeals or superstitious calls to the witchy ways of the oppressed. New evidence needed to be developed to reinforce existing ideologies and systems. Thus, alongside scientific discoveries that remain relevant today, such as Galileo's exploration of the galaxies with his improvements to the telescope in the seventeenth century or

Linnaeus' revolutionary new taxonomy for classifying nature in the eighteenth century, we also see the introduction of eugenics, scientific racism, and appeals to nature as a means to keep hierarchies of domination intact. In other words, much like religion or magic, appeals to science can be used to dispel myths or to reinforce them. From the vantage of the early twenty-first century, there remains confusion as to what "the science" says about breastfeeding, though lactivists would dispute this vehemently (Joan Wolf 2013). Digging beneath the surface of breastfeeding promotion we can see that a lot of "scientific" claims are more ideological or even theological than evidence based. In fact, breastfeeding, viewed as a cultural and social practice, has the potential to challenge some of our most fundamental assumptions about science, nature, and *Mammalia* in general.

What Is Science?

Breastfeeding is often framed as natural and as scientifically proven to be better for babies. To deny "the science," as discussed in chapter 2, is to incite anger and accusations of being in the pocket of big formula or to be likened to a Holocaust denier (Joan Wolf 2013). However, this reflects a misunderstanding of how science works. Although science studies nature, science does not speak for nature. Scientific inquiry is a tool for excavating evidence, not an arbiter of right and wrong. Science can determine the "best-ness" of something about as well as a hammer can decide if the drapes go with the loveseat. So, first, let's pause to think about what science is and what it is not.

Sociologist Rodney Stark offers a helpful definition of science as "a method utilized in organized efforts to explain nature, always subject to modifications and corrections through systematic observations" (2001, 103). In this way, science is distinct from magic, religion, and empiricism in that science alone involves both theory and research – that is, both observation and testing theories that might explain what has been observed. Magic and empiricism involve trial and error, and observation, but no theory. Religion involves theory and perhaps observation, but no empirical testing.

A significant difference between magical or religious thinking and science is that practitioners of the former try to *prove* their theories, whereas those doing the latter seek to *disprove* theirs. This process of disproving is referred to as empirical falsification. In the social sciences, empirical falsification is typically associated with the work of mid-twentieth-century philosopher of science Karl Popper, who contributed to the development of positivism in the social sciences. This insistence that theories be able to withstand scientific investigation was a major shift in the discipline of sociology. Though there is variation in the degree to which any particular sociologist subscribes to Popperian positivism, the legacy of his theorizing, along with the political action of William Fielding Ogburn (Laslett 1990), is that deductive, empirical science is the predominant paradigm in American sociology today, although qualitative feminist and other critical and Marxist perspectives retain a significant foothold among sociologists, especially outside the United States. Within health sciences and medicine and the other natural or "hard" sciences, positivism is practically the only epistemology employed – so much so that they just call it "science."

To understand science (including positivist social science), it is important to understand the difference between deductive and inductive logic. Within inductive logic, one makes repeated observations from which universal conclusions are drawn. For example, if every day I see that the sun comes up, I can logically induce that the sun will rise again tomorrow. However, just because something occurs repeatedly, there is no guarantee that it will occur again. As Popper writes, "no matter how many instances of white swans we may have observed, this does not justify the conclusion that all swans are white" ([1959] 2005, 4).

As such, he advocates for the use of methods that allow for logical *deduction*, because deductive logic does allow one to draw accurate universal conclusions, as long as the premises within the logic are true. An example of deductive logic might be the following:

(a) All birds have feathers.
(b) Swans are birds.
(c) Therefore, swans have feathers.

As long as (a) and (b) are true, (c) must also be true. The challenge, then, is in figuring out whether (a) and (b) are true. Since mere observation of birds cannot guarantee that all birds have feathers, one should try to find cases of birds that do not have feathers. Once a featherless bird is found, one's theory falls apart, but the science is stronger. We have more evidence to build into new deductive theories. Thus, empirical falsification – the methodology of science – is the process of trying to falsify our theories through rigorous and repeated testing. Empirical falsification is argued to be superior to making inferences because it seeks to establish what is, rather than what might be. In the words of Stark,

> Not only do systematic observations yield empirical generalizations that can prompt the construction of theories, far more important is that any scientific theory is subject to contraction by observations. As noted, a scientific theory predicts and prohibits certain observable states of affairs. It says, this is what must occur, and this is what may not occur. When these predictions and prohibitions are not consistent with the relevant observations it is necessary to reject or revise that theory. It is by being able to falsify theories that science makes progress. By ruthlessly weeding out theories that fail, or which are less efficient or precise, we gain confidence in those that continue to survive confrontations with the facts ... Just as vulnerability to falsification is the primary scientific virtue, it is a primary weakness of magic. It is assumed that scientific "truths" are provisional, subject to future rejection or revision, but this is not the assumption on which magic rests. When magic fails, as it often does, this seldom inspires magicians to revise, but merely to try again, and again. (2001, 113–14)

Thus, science can be distinguished from magic or religion in terms of the scientists' lack of faith in their claims compared with the absolute faith of magicians and theologians in theirs. Science cannot exist if scientists adhere to their claims as a matter of faith.

What Is Nature?

Although not all sociologists see themselves as scientists, those who do are following in the footsteps of Émile Durkheim, who first introduced science as a means to study social life in the late nineteenth century. Durkheim published multiple works to demonstrate that we can study social life in the same ways that a biologist can study natural life: through careful measurement of data. For instance, in one of his key works, *Suicide*, Durkheim ([1897] 2005) studied suicide as a product of social conditions and not merely individual pathologies, by using data on regional suicide rates in France to understand how the suicide rate differed depending on local economic or social conditions. In this way, sociologists tend not to study elements of social life that cannot be measured. We might explore religious practices, but we would not treat a religious text as the word of God.

Similarly, we avoid answering our research questions on the grounds that something is "natural" or "what nature intended." Nature does not have much of a place in sociological explanations, not only because we can't really measure what's "natural" but also because sociologists generally agree that a large majority of social processes, social life, social facts, and so forth are a construction. This idea is typically credited to Berger and Luckmann, who wrote, "*Society is a human product. Society is an objective reality. Man is a social product*" (1966, 79; their italics). What we as sociologists do is to try to uncover the ways in which what we think of as reality came to be and the elements of social life that we hold to be so normal or so "natural" that they seem inevitable.

In this way, sociology rejects "nature" as an explanation because our goal is to understand the reasons behind social constructions. Whereas positivist sociologists are interested in understanding these social constructions for the sake of pure knowledge, *critical* sociologists, seek to uncover these social structures as a means to critique and change them. If we see social inequality or racism or another factor of social life that causes harm, the idea that the situation is "natural" would suggest that nothing can be done to change it. Similarly, if something is viewed as "unnatural," then coming to see it as natural can have significant implications for people's lives. Before Berger and Luckmann, in 1928 William Isaac Thomas and Dorothy Swaine Thomas developed the "Thomas Theorem," which states that if people "define situations as real they become real in their consequences" ([1928] 1938, 572). This raises important questions: If people believe that something is natural, what are the consequences of this belief? Who gets to decide if something is natural? Who benefits from certain activities or patterns being defined as natural? In sociology, we typically see that those with more power can use that power to define what's natural, and typically they define what's natural in ways that benefit themselves.

What Could Be More Natural Than Breastfeeding?

There is no question that lactation is a biological function of the human body that has been essential to human survival. Breastfeeding has been necessary not only in meeting babies' nutritional needs but also, according to primatologists, in allowing humans to evolve from tree-swinging primates into bipedal humans who could use language (Huber 2007). That said, medical ethicists Jessica Martucci and Anne Barnhill (2016) published a paper in the journal *Pediatrics* suggesting that public health promotion should avoid using claims to nature because such appeals have unintended consequences for other public health initiatives. Specifically, they point out that claiming that "natural" things are better could discourage parents from getting their children vaccinated, since vaccines are manufactured and not found in nature. Martucci and Barnhill write,

> The idea of the "natural" evokes a sense of purity, goodness, and harmlessness. Meanwhile, synthetic substances, products, and technologies produced by industry (notably, vaccines) are seen as "unnatural" and often arouse suspicion and distrust. Part of this value system is the perception that what's natural is safer, healthier, and less risky. This embrace of the "natural" over the "unnatural" appears in a variety of contemporary scientific and medical issues beyond vaccination, including rejection of genetically modified foods, a preference for organic over conventionally grown foods, and rejection of assisted reproductive technologies, as well as concerns over environmental toxins and water fluoridation. Much of the interest in complementary and alternative medicines also hinges on "ideas of natural techniques as safer, gentler and benign." (2)

Martucci and Barnhill (2016) assert that arguments for the benefits of something based on its "naturalness" are rooted in values and beliefs rather than in science. Although logical, their argument incited some controversy, including an outraged discussion of their work by conservative Fox News commentator Tucker Carlson on 15 October 2017 (Etienne 2017). He brought in a self-described feminist (*cum* straw man) to stumble around trying to defend the ideas, grimacing at her every word. Through squinted eyes and with an exasperated tone, he asked, "If breastfeeding is not natural, what is natural?" What was most interesting to me about his response is that he cared so much. Why was he so mad at the suggestion that breastfeeding isn't natural? Is it possible that power structures that benefit Carlson are being challenged with the assertion that breast may not be best? Again, as Berger and Luckmann pointed out back in 1966, "Generally speaking, in situations where there is competition between different reality-defining agencies, all sorts of secondary-group relationships with the competitors may be tolerated, as long as there are firmly established primary-group relationships within which one reality is on-goingly reaffirmed against the competitors" (172). In other words, when a social group is more firmly established as dominant, this group will not tolerate any challenges to the existing social order. And, infant feeding has been tied more closely to the social roles and relative power allocated to women and men than just about any other mammalian behaviour.

The problem with the social construction of maternal breastfeeding as "natural" is that this claim implies that it is the *only* natural way to feed or nurture infants. Scientifically speaking, this is not the case. Allomater-nal nursing, in which mothers feed other women's babies, was common among the hunters and gatherers (Hewlett and Winn 2014) and is seen across at least one hundred mammalian species (Packer, Lewis, and Pusey 1992). According to anthropologists Barry S. Hewlett and Steve Winn (2014), allomaternal nursing was said to characterize "over 90% of modern Homo sapiens history," and in their review of the electronic Human Re-lations Area Files database, they found that allomaternal nursing "existed in 97 of 104 cultures with ethnographic data." Further, the "natural" act of shared breastfeeding is found among other "cooperative breeders" such as tufted capuchin monkeys and sperm whales (200).

Anthropologist Sarah Blaffer Hrdy points out that "throughout the Animal Kingdom, and most especially in species that produce immobile, utterly helpless babies that need a lot of maternal care (the way baby pri-mates do), infants exude potent signals, captivating the susceptible. Related or not, infants can be powerful sensory traps" (2009, 211). These "sensory traps" (209) can be downright addictive, causing mothers to crave access to their babies. In experiments with lactating rats, when rat mothers were given "a choice between pushing a lever that would administer cocaine or one that would cause pups to tumble one after another into her cage, the mother filled her cage with pups" (213). She goes on to note that most of these studies used laboratory rats, mice, or voles, but rhesus macaques and humans have been shown to experience the same phenomenon.

Indeed, when members of Eric Keverne's lab at the University of Cambridge chemically blocked the action of endogenous opioids, maternal responsiveness to infants declined. Infants have similarly rewarding effects on human mothers. It should not be surprising that studies using MRIs show activation of dopamine-associated reward centers in the brains of first-time human mothers when they look at photographs of their smiling infant. Any number of cues would probably have a similar effect – suckling, soft coos, a familiar baby's chuckle, the seductive smells emitted from the glands on her baby's scalp. (213)

Although most research has been carried out on mothers, Hrdy (2009) observes that birth mothers are not the only ones to get a hormonal hit of dopamine or oxytocin, the pleasure-releasing hormones, when presented with an intoxicating baby. Across mammals where alloparenting is carried out,

> juveniles and subadult females who have never been pregnant or given birth also spontaneously respond to infants, huddling over pups to keep them warm. In infant-sharing primates such as langurs, these females exhibit irrepressible urges to sniff, touch, cuddle, and repeatedly take and carry new babies. In marmosets and tamarins, males – especially those with prior caretaking experience – also eagerly respond to infant vocalization and other cues, and they may be even more eager than females are to caretake ...
>
> In both marmosets and men, males who engage in a lot of care have higher prolactin levels than males who do not. Other species characterized by nurturing males include California mice, Mongolian gerbils, African meerkats, and Djungerian hamsters. The inclination to care for infants derives from ancient and fairly universal physiological systems that are normally operational only in mothers. In these species, however, nurturing tendencies get switched on in males as well. (213–14)

According to Hrdy, this intoxicating quality of babies is an evolutionary adaptation that encourages others to pass them around, thereby allowing mothers to reproduce more frequently and lowering infant mortality, since babies can rely on more than just one person for their every need. This suggests that what babies need is *not* just one parent who can do and be everything for them but a sense that they "will be cared for no matter what" (2009, 119). As in several other mammalian species, mothers are not the only humans whose biological drives urge them to respond to babies – theirs, or someone else's.

Despite clear scientific evidence of men's capacity for caregiving, rarely is "nature" used as a justification for why men should give care. Rarer still are men encouraged to breastfeed, despite evidence of their capacity to give milk (Kunz and Hosken 2009). All human beings are born with nipples and milk ducts regardless of their assigned or chosen sex. The extent to which cisgender men could sustain a newborn life is unknown, but there seems to be close to zero interest in exploring the potential of fathers' nipples to provide basic soothing to babies. One might think this idea would have caught on, given that lactivists have promoted the now debunked notion that pacifiers should not be used for the first month of life for fear of causing nipple confusion (O'Connor et al. 2009).

Hewlett (1989) discusses the Aka pygmy tribe in northern Congo, where men commonly nurse or suckle babies while mothers go out to hunt. In this society, parenting is shared fully equally and there is no stigma to nurturing babies; it is viewed as work for all. More recent research using qualitative interviews found "that fathers are more likely to sing or dance with the infant or give her water before offering his breasts. Mothers said fathers' nipples were too small and the infants preferred the larger nipples of their grandmothers" (Hewlett and Winn 2014, 205). However, the authors note that previous research studies "observed more Aka and Bofi infants on the breasts of their fathers than on the breasts of adolescent females" (210). Unclear is whether fathers in this culture serve as much more than pacifiers, regardless of their capacity to produce milk.

In an opinion piece in the journal *Trends in Ecology and Evolution*, conservation biologists Thomas H. Kunz and David J. Hosken (2009) explore why lactation has typically been restricted to females, following the discovery of milk-producing males in two species of Old World fruit bats in Malaysia (Francis et al. 1994) and Papua New Guinea (Bonaccorso 1998). Kunz and Hosken (2009) explain that in primates, including humans, the nipples of male and female mammals develop in the same way from birth until males get a shot of androgens (male hormones) at puberty. Interestingly, the biological process that leads to lactation after birth can be triggered in the absence of childbirth taking place. During pregnancy, lactation is inhibited by high levels of estrogen and progesterone, which take a sharp drop postpartum in order to signal to the pituitary that prolactin can be released, thereby causing milk to be released. (This sudden hormonal drop also explains why, as my midwife presciently told me, many women spend the first day their milk comes in crying.) What further stimulates the production of prolactin is the suckling by the baby. This is why lactation can be induced in women who have never given birth or who gave birth a long time ago (Kunz and Hosken 2009), including the allomaternal nursing grandmothers mentioned above.

Kunz and Hosken (2009) identify a number of documented cases of human and other mammalian males who have been found to produce milk, including Holocaust survivors who had experienced extreme malnutrition that damaged their endocrine systems and male sheep that ate grasses high in compounds similar to endogenous estrogens. With so little research into induced male lactation, we know very little about what possibilities might exist for men to sustain an infant with adequate nutrition, although this curiosity is not new. According to historian Londa Schiebinger, eighteenth-century naturalists like Carl Linnaeus were interested in exploring men's capacity to lactate, although she dismisses the concept as "fanciful":

> The fanciful notion that males are, indeed, capable of producing
> milk was popular among naturalists. Aristotle had considered it
> an omen of extraordinary good fortune when a male goat pro-
> duced milk in such quantities that cheese could be made from it.
> Eighteenth-century naturalists reported the secretion of a fatty
> milky substance – "witch's milk" – from the breasts of male as well as
> female newborns. [Georges-Louis Leclerc, the Comte de] Buffon re-
> lated many examples of the male breast filling with milk at the onset
> of puberty. A boy of fifteen, for example, pressed from one of his
> breasts more than a spoonful of "true" milk. John Hunter offered the
> example of a father who nursed his eight children. This man began
> nursing when his wife was unable to satisfy a set of twins. "To soothe
> the cries of the male child," Hunter wrote, "the father applied his left
> nipple to the infant's mouth, who drew milk from it in such quantity
> as to be nursed in perfectly good health." (The father also shared
> with his wife all other domestic duties.) Considering milk produc-
> tion within the bounds of normal male physiology, Hunter dutifully
> noted that the man "was not a hermaphrodite." (1993, 389)

Still, in a letter to the editor responding to Kunz and Hosken's (2009) article, Racey, Peaker, and Racey point out that "galactorrhoea is not lactation," stating that "in medical science, male nipple discharge is termed 'galactorrhoea' and the growth of male breast tissue 'gynecomastia.' In humans, the most common presentation of male galactorrhea and gynecomastia is a physiological by-product of hormonal change in puberty and is transient" (2009, 354). This may explain why, when I excitedly reported to a large undergraduate sociology class I was teaching that men can lactate, three students said something along the lines of "Yeah, so what? I knew three guys in high school who could do that and would show everyone at parties." Call me shocked.

Regardless of whether male "lactation" can be more than a party trick, I find the lack of attention to possible uses for the male nipple – a *natural* part of the male body – telling. In an early version of the paper my colleague Mary C. Noonan and I eventually published in the *American Sociological Review*, we discussed the possibility of male lactation as a solution to the negative impact on wages experienced by women who breastfeed for more than six months (Rippeyoung and Noonan 2012b). The suggestion was dismissed by one reviewer, who wrote, "Women face numerous constraints on their infant feeding choices depending on their social location. Social change in these areas is much more relevant than the consideration of male breastfeeding." I don't entirely disagree with this reviewer, and we removed most of our discussion of this topic from the article. Clearly, getting male or female partners to induce lactation does nothing to address the needs of single mothers or mothers with abusive spouses (Blum 1999). The battle to get men on board as breastfeeders may also be a steep hill to die on.

On a personal note, when I suggested to my own husband that he try to breastfeed our newborn son, he was adamantly opposed, saying it was just "weird." My older sons have also affirmed that there is no way they will ever try such a thing. Despite their protestations, there were moments when my last baby, twelve and fifteen years younger than my older boys, would hungrily try to latch on to whoever happened to be holding him, and I enjoyed seeing these guys' curious facial expressions when it occurred.

There have also been recent discussions of "chestfeeding" by transgender men (that is, men assigned female at birth) who give birth, but even that has caused considerable controversy. In 2012, Canadian trans-dad Trevor MacDonald was denied the opportunity to be a La Leche leader for a queer breastfeeding support group he wanted to organize. After successfully chestfeeding his birth child with much support from La Leche League, MacDonald wanted to become a La Leche leader to help support other LGBTQ parents. La Leche League first rejected his request on the grounds that the organization had been established for "mother-to-mother" support, which did not allow for father-led support. It since changed its policy, eventually making MacDonald a leader (Tapper 2014). The La Leche League Canada website now notes, under the header "Who we are," that

"La Leche League Canada is a registered nonprofit that provides mother-to-mother/parent-to-parent/peer support for pregnant women, new parents and beyond. We are parents like you who have breastfed or chestfed our own children and now volunteer to support others to reach their goals" ("La Leche League Canada" n.d.).

Although chest- or breastfeeding by men may sound "weird," another taboo, wet-nursing, was at one time quite common. What is odd today may be common practice among our sons in the future. And, even if addressing women's barriers to breastfeeding might be a more pressing concern than addressing men's barriers to engaging in the practice, the mere possibility that men can breastfeed challenges our notions of what is natural or necessary. Further, it highlights the unequal attention given to policies that encourage women's "natural" tendencies or capacities to nurture relative to men's.

Introducing *Mammalia*

Considering that male nursing has been given such short shrift, one might wonder why it was decided to call us mammals, given the common practice of centring men in science. As Schiebinger points out, "the class *Mammalia* was the only one of [the] major zoological divisions to focus on reproductive organs and the only term to highlight a characteristic associated primarily with the female" (1993, 384). This is especially puzzling given that not all members of the class *Mammalia* were originally thought to breastfeed. Monotremes, for example, such as the platypus or echidna, have no nipples, though they do have mammary glands that lactate. They just ooze milk through pores in mothers' bellies that their babies lap up (Schiebinger 1993). Given these anomalous animals, the fact that functional mammary glands were assumed to be unique to women, and that there are other traits we share with our mammal brethren, there is something curious about the fact that the father of our current taxonomic system, Swedish botanist Carolus Linnaeus, would have made breastfeeding the defining characteristic of our species in the tenth edition of *Systema Naturae*, in 1758. Schiebinger notes that there were numerous other options for organizing the species that he could have gone with and that "*Lactentia* or *Sugentia* (both meaning 'the suckling ones') would have better universalized the term, since male as well as female young suckle at their mothers' breasts" (392). As such, she writes, "because Linnaeus had choices, I suggest that his focus on the breast responded to broader cultural and political trends" (393).

Prior to Linnaeus' taxonomy, there were all kinds of competing systems for organizing and classifying living organisms. For over two thousand years, most mammals, not including humans, were referred to as quadrupeds, defined as an animal on four feet. Aristotle and the naturalists who followed came up with numerous variations on this taxonomy although all retained the "quadruped" terminology until British naturalist John Ray (1627–1705) came along and noticed that aquatic animals like dolphins are more similar to mammals than to fish in important ways, though they lack four feet. Such changes took decades to be fully accepted, and Linneaus himself included "quadruped" in the first edition of his *Systema Naturae* (1735). The notion that humans would be in the same taxonomic category as animals was seen as both outrageous and heresy, given that "Holy Scripture, after all, clearly taught that man was created in God's image" (Schiebinger 1993, 386). Linneaus finally accepted the grouping of humans with animals when he settled on the term *Mammalia* in 1758, with the defence that "even if his critics did not believe that humans originally walked on all fours, surely every man born of woman must admit that he was nourished by his mother's milk" (387). Though the term had detractors, it nonetheless was hugely popular and quickly stuck.

Although one might see this as a kind of woman-centred or feminist valuing of women's role in maintaining the human species, Schiebinger cautions against so optimistic an interpretation:

> It is important to note, however, that in the same volume in which Linnaeus introduced the term *Mammalia,* he also introduced the name *Homo sapiens*. This term, "man of wisdom," was used to distinguish humans from other primates (apes, lemurs, and bats, for example). In the language of taxonomy, *sapiens* is what is known as a "trivial" name. (Linnaeus at one point pondered the choice of the name *Homo diurnus,* designed to contrast with *Homo nocturnus*.) From a historical point of view, however, the choice of the term *sapiens* is highly significant. "Man" had traditionally been distinguished from animals by his reason; the medieval apposition, *animal rationale*, proclaimed his uniqueness. Thus, within Linnaean terminology, a female characteristic (the lactating mamma) ties humans to brutes, while a traditionally male characteristic (reason) marks our separateness. (1993, 393–4)

Linneaus found a receptive audience for his new taxonomy. As Schiebinger observes,

> His scientific vision arose alongside important political trends in the eighteenth century – the restructuring of both child care and women's lives as mothers, wives, and citizens. The stress he placed on the naturalness of a mother giving suck to her young reinforced the social movement's undermining the public power of women and attaching a new value to mothering. Despite the Enlightenment credo that all "men" were by nature equal, middle-class women were not to become fully enfranchised citizens or professionals in the state but newly empowered mothers within the home.
>
> Most directly, Linnaeus joined the campaign to abolish the ancient custom of wet nursing. (1993, 404)

Although these concepts were shaped by thousands of years of patriarchal ideology, they were newly framed in terms of both nature and science. The emphasis on women's breastfeeding and men's reason in this taxonomy also coincided with the takeover of medicine by male gynecologists and obstetricians who replaced women midwives, the birth attendants women had relied on since humans evolved from primates (Huber 2007).

Scientific classification was used to reinforce social constructions not only of gender but also of race. According to anthropologists Audrey Smedley and Brian Smedley (2005), race as a concept was invented as a means to offer scientific justification for slavery. Scientists would use physical characteristics typical of people from African colonies to make claims about internal or personality traits. Thus, the colour of one's skin or the measurements of specific body parts were said to be indicative of superiority, inferiority, or pathology. At the intersection of these racist and patriarchal notions of breastfeeding was the scientific claim that Black and White women had different natural capacities for breastfeeding. According to historians Emily West and R.J. Knight,

> European colonial travelers to West Africa frequently commented on black women's breasts as large and droopy and compared them to goats' udders. According to Jennifer L. Morgan, early European travelers typically commented that West African women's breasts were long, enabling women to suckle their infants over their shoulders. Referring to these black African women's breasts as *dugges* – an

archaic word that meant either a woman's breast or animal's teat – also "connoted a brute animality." (2017, 39–40)

This linkage of Black women to brute animals thus suggested that childbirth and nursing were somehow easier for Black women and that they were also better suited to hard manual labour than were White women. As Dorothy Roberts writes, in her now classic book *Killing the Black Body*,

> The essence of Black women's experience during slavery was the brutal denial of autonomy over reproduction. Female slaves were commercially valuable to their masters not only for their labor, but also for their ability to produce more slaves. The law made slave women's children the property of the slaveowner. White masters therefore could increase their wealth by controlling their slaves' reproductive capacity. With owners expecting natural multiplication to generate as much as 5 to 6 percent of their profit, they had a strong incentive to maximize their slaves' fertility ... Slave births and deaths were not recorded in the family Bible but in the slaveholder's business ledger. ([1997] 2017, 24)

This control extended not only to the theft of Black women's babies but also to selective breeding programs in which the strongest enslaved men were forced to share beds and have sex with enslaved women in the hopes of creating superior "stock" to sell at market. Infertile enslaved women would be beaten or killed for the crime of not producing saleable babies for their masters. One result of the valuing of enslaved Black women for their reproductive labour and their physical labour, combined with a poor understanding of prenatal health (Roberts [1997] 2014), led to many Black women being forced to labour in the fields while pregnant and soon after the birth of their child. According to West and Knight (2017), for some slaves this meant having their child taken from them to be wet-nursed by another slave or, occasionally, by the White mistress of the house.

Enslaved African women were exploited not only by White male elites for free reproductive labour but also by White women as a means "to manipulate enslaved women's motherhood for slaveholders' own ends" (West and Knight 2017, 37). Whereas in Europe, elite mothers typically had to pay for the services of a wet nurse, in the antebellum South, slave-holding mistresses were able to procure the service for "free from [their] own chattel"

(39). Although male slaveholders were technically the ones in command of such systems, their White wives were eager to procure the services of a "free" wet nurse to liberate themselves from the tiring and sometimes painful work of nursing a baby around the clock. White women also justified their use of enslaved wet nurses in terms of convenience, freeing them to feel not "'tied to the place' and to her demanding baby's beck and call" and helping them avoid having their "breast to be flat" (53). The greater privilege and freedom afforded to White women through the usage of Black women's bodies led to changes in how housework and motherhood were valued. As West and Knight write,

> White women's relative position of power and privilege compared with their enslaved women permitted them (unlike female slaves) to make their own decisions about whether to breast-feed their own children. They acted as "mother-managers" within their homes, possessing the power to delegate the most taxing and least desirable elements of motherhood to their slaves, including wet-nursing, infant and child care, and caring for the elderly. They manipulated the motherhood of enslaved women for their own ends. (2017, 53–4)

Within the context of slavery and the period immediately following, the association between nature and breastfeeding was decidedly a negative one. Viewed as a behaviour of animals, the practice was to be avoided not only by White men but also by affluent White women. Though in other cultures and eras breastfeeding has been constructed as a communal responsibility or even an experience of the Divine, women elites of the seventeenth and eighteenth centuries saw it as something to be avoided if possible.

But, C'mon, Isn't Biology a Thing?

In her book *On the Origins of Gender Inequality*, sociologist Joan Huber critiques sociological and anthropological approaches to gender inequality that fail to consider biological realities, writing that "the idea that human values and customs are a purely social construction is a roadmap to a dead end. Causal analysis must be based on variables rooted in the real world (e.g., soil fertility, climate, technology, terrain) that offer differentiating average conditions in which people employ routines adapted to local conditions and the resources that make the routines practical" (2007,

95). While acknowledging that much of the biological sciences were highly androcentric and biased against women for many years, she argues that understanding why men came to dominate nearly all human societies in nearly all contexts requires us to grapple with the biological and environmental realities of human life. She locates lactation as the root cause of gender inequality, given its demands on women's bodies and the necessity of breastfeeding to human survival.

Although I agree with Huber that breastfeeding places enormous burdens on women who breastfeed, I would argue that biological and evolutionary realities shape not only how infants are fed but also the impulse to protect the welfare of babies over the welfare of mothers. As discussed above, there is plenty of evidence that human survival has depended on cooperation in the raising of infants and children (Hrdy 2009). While social scientists have explored these ideas primarily from a perspective of self-interest or social functioning, there is much to be learned from evolutionary biologists about infant feeding and caring. A question that occurred to me in this research is why international development agencies have been so focused on saving babies but less interested in saving women and even less in saving men. Where do we get the idea of "women and children first"? Is this historical chivalry simply a result of power grabs?

As shown in the experiments with rats, macaques, and humans discussed by Hrdy (2009), an element of our evolutionary wiring seems to make humans want to save and protect things that are cute. I personally observed my youngest son kiss images of cute kittens, puppies, and babies in books and videos at least as young as twenty months old, but he never had the same reaction to images of old men or even beloved fire trucks and dinosaurs. So, what is it that would lead this child to feel a need to express love to images of babies? This is not to deny misogyny or the role of power in how societies are organized, but rather to add another piece of the puzzle in answering the question of why our society is ordered as it is. Part of what makes breastfeeding important for social scientists to explore is the way in which the practice challenges us to tease out the "real" from the social constructions – the inevitable from the changeable.

Joan Huber (2007) offers a useful survey on the history of infant feeding practices that offers some possible answers to these questions. According to her review of the literature, about five million years ago primates began to evolve into hominids who could walk on two feet. A few million years later they began to use speech. For both of these things to occur, changes in the composition of the human body were required: the human pelvis had to shrink to make it easier to walk on two legs, while at the same time the bigger brain required for speech also required a larger pelvis in women to make vaginal birth possible. The solution to this evolutionary trade-off was that for human infants to be small enough to fit through the birth canal, we needed to be born less developed than our primate cousins. Citing Lancaster (1985), Huber points out,

> At birth, a human infant's brain is relatively smaller in proportion to its adult size than in any closely related primate: 23 percent of adult size in a human compared to 45 percent in the chimpanzee and 68 percent in the rhesus monkey. In six or seven months the human brain has grown to 45 percent of adult size. By the fourth year, it is 95 percent of adult size, the usual age of weaning among foragers. (2007, 69)

Additionally, our bipedalism also meant that the human birth canal took a different shape than the birth canal of our simian ancestors. Whereas the breadths of quadrupedal mammals' heads match those of their mothers' birth canals, as Huber writes,

> The evolution of bipedalism twisted the human birth canal in the middle so that the entrance is broadest side to side while the exit is broadest front to back ... The passage of the infant's broad, rigid shoulders through the mother's bony pelvis requires that the infant's chin be pressed against its throat instead of tilted backwards or extended, like the monkey's. The coupling of this flexion with the restructured bony birth canal requires that the human infant undergo a series of rotations to pass through the birth canal without hindrance. (Huber 2007, 69–70)

Consequently, this new design means that whereas all other mammal mothers can birth alone, human mothers need assistance to give birth. Because the rotations at birth lead an infant to face their mother's back, with their chin tucked under, the mother is unable "to reach down and clear a breathing passageway for it or to remove the cord from around its neck should the cord be interfering with breathing or continued emergence" (70). Human babies are at greater risk of injury if mothers try to guide the baby out of the birth canal owing to the awkward positioning of the baby relative to the mother's eyes and arms. These evolutionary changes in the human body mean that human babies are born far needier and more help-less for longer periods than any other mammal. This neediness also had the consequence of increasing the amount of work that mothers would have to do, most notably in terms of a far longer period of dependence on caregivers for food.

Although lactation supported human survival, breastfeeding practices have evolved over the past forty thousand or more years. According to Huber, "throughout human history an infant was suckled at intervals of about 15 minutes during the day and less often at night for its first two years, then less often day and night for another two years" (2007, 2). This is far different from the current general guidelines to feed infants every two to three hours. This around-the-clock breastfeeding for four years is what Huber claims explains the nearly universal pattern of male domin-ance across time and space around the globe. Mothers, tied to their babies because of their need to be fed so frequently, were not able to venture away from their territories to build alliances and gather resources to the extent that men could. Huber's argument – that lactation is the root cause of gender inequality – is supported by the observation that by and large, women have only been able to enter political, economic, and social life in large numbers since suitable milk substitutes were introduced into the market early in the twentieth century (Huber 2007; Albanesi and Olivetti 2016). Until then, without mothers' work breastfeeding, babies (indeed, the entire human race) would have died.

Though breastfeeding has been essential to human evolution, as fem-inist breastfeeding advocate Bernice Hausman (2003) points out, the "breast is best/most natural" rhetoric used by breastfeeding proponents often misrepresents how evolution works. In a critique of anthropologist Kathy Dettwyler's (1995) argument in favour of extended breastfeeding, Hausman challenges the relevance of early hominid feeding patterns to the choices we make today. Dettwyler, like many breastfeeding advocates, claims that breastfeeding ensures "optimal development" (134) and helps children "thrive" (134) especially when practised in a manner similar to that of our hominid ancestors. However, Hausman (2003) points out that in contrast to technologies, which do have the capacity to improve life ex-periences and outcomes, evolutionary processes are about adaptation to one's environment, not about creating the perfect or best solution. Human evolution involves trade-offs – walking on two legs opened up huge possi-bilities for movement and growth but led to backaches and difficulties with childbirth; speech made communication and growth possible but also increased the risk of choking while eating.

Put another way, our early human history need not define us. Although breastfeeding was important to humans becoming bipedal, it does not necessarily follow that humans must continue to breastfeed any more than we should feel obligated to follow other practices of early humans. Early humans did not have computers on which to write blogs about the benefits of breastfeeding, but that is hardly a reason to impede lactivists' access to Blogger. Cancer can be wired into our DNA but that doesn't mean we don't seek a cure for it. Poison ivy is natural, but we don't want it in our backyards.

As the evidence discussed in this chapter shows, it is infant feeding and caregiving that has kept our species alive, not particular manners of carry-ing out these activities. Ascribing value to the practice on the basis that it is natural would be akin to ascribing value to replacing one's cooking utensils with rocks. It is an option, but it might not work for everyone. In a later chapter I will explore scientific studies on the benefits of breast milk, but the important point here is that science examines evidence and de-velops theories – it does not tell us what to do. Telling other people how to feed their babies based on an interpretation of what is natural is a political, not a scientific, act. As will be seen in the next chapter, claims about what nature can teach us about the responsibilities of women have a long and storied history, flourishing most famously in the work of Enlightenment political philosopher Jean-Jacques Rousseau.

6 Enlightened Breasts

Would you restore all men to their primal duties, begin with the mothers; the results will surprise you. Every evil follows in the train of this first sin; the whole moral order is disturbed, nature is quenched in every breast, the home becomes gloomy, the spectacle of a young family no longer stirs the husband's love and the stranger's reverence. The mother whose children are out of sight wins scanty esteem; there is no home life, the ties of nature are not strengthened by those of habit; fathers, mothers, children, brothers, and sisters cease to exist. They are almost strangers; how should they love one another? Each thinks of himself first. When the home is a gloomy solitude pleasure will be sought elsewhere.

But when mothers deign to nurse their own children, then will be a reform in morals; natural feeling will revive in every heart; there will be no lack of citizens for the state; this first step by itself will restore mutual affection. The charms of home are the best antidote to vice. The noisy play of children, which we thought so trying, becomes a delight; mother and father rely more on each other and grow dearer to one another; the marriage tie is strengthened. In the cheerful home life the mother finds her sweetest duties and the father his pleasantest recreation. Thus the cure of this one evil would work a wide-spread reformation; nature would regain her rights. When women become good mothers, men will be good husbands and fathers.

Jean-Jacques Rousseau, *Émile*

Alongside the flourishing of scientific inquiry (Stark 2001), the seventeenth- and eighteenth-century European Enlightenment was revolutionary in spirit and in actual fact of political change. Compared with the witch hunts of the Middle Ages, a certain kind of social stability was found in the new capitalist system of the West, although social unrest did not disappear. Philosophical debates raged throughout Europe and the colonies as intellectuals argued the possibilities of social and political structures that could put an end to monarchical rule, culminating in the American and French Revolutions of 1776 and 1789, respectively. Within such debates, a fundamental question was how to balance human freedom with state authority, especially if a society no longer had a king to make all the rules. Contained within this question were the respective roles and rights of women and men.

Many philosophers, most famously the Swiss philosopher Jean-Jacques Rousseau, concluded that women's purpose was to control and discipline men's more wild natures. One basis for Rousseau's claims was women's capacity to breastfeed. In fact, to Rousseau, mothers' breastfeeding of their own children was a civic duty necessary for the maintenance of a properly functioning society. Unlike other gendered prescriptions that kept women away from public life (such as the claim of women's inferior capacity to reason), Rousseau's idealization of the importance of breastfeeding was an idea that even pre-feminist icons of the day like Mary Wollstonecraft could get on board with.

Morality without God

After thousands of years of religion and magic being used to address moral questions, the introduction of science in the early Enlightenment posed a rather puzzling dilemma to philosophers. If science relies on empirical falsification over faith in God, and if the goal of science is to prove one's claims wrong rather than right, science would seem to be entirely useless for providing answers to moral questions. As outlined in the previous chapter, science can offer evidence to help us make decisions based on our moral beliefs, but science alone can never answer what one should do or how one ought to feel about a particular issue. At the same time, if science has undermined reliance on God as the foundation for moral theorizing how are those in a secular, modernizing society to answer moral questions? As Stark writes, "Of course, as noted, any number of moral rules can be *asserted* on purely secular grounds. And they can be enforced, given sufficient group solidarity." He continues, "But a crucial philosophical problem persists: lacking the legitimacy provided by divine will, how is it possible to *justify* moral rules, to prevent them from being seen as arbitrary, provisional, and subject to individual choice?" (2001, 113).

One solution that emerged in the seventeenth- and eighteenth-century thinking of John Locke, Montesquieu, and Jean-Jacques Rousseau, among others, was to resolve moral dilemmas through appeals to nature. Through the guise of science, these philosophers could make moral claims about "proven" natural truths while also referencing the Bible, logic, and common sense. Fundamentally, these influential Enlightenment philosophers sought political goals, including overthrowing monarchical rule and creating a political system in which men could be ensured their rights to life, liberty, property, and the pursuit of happiness – creating what we today call classical liberalism. Monarchies are a political structure that are said to be divinely ordered, and therefore to attack a king or queen would be to attack the religion that gave them their authority. Therefore, for thinkers like Rousseau in Europe or Thomas Jefferson in the United States to advocate for societies free from monarchical rule, they needed to demonstrate how moral order could be maintained without religion. To reject the notion of kings having a divine right to rule and an exclusive connection with God, their answer was that "man" could be self-determining because nature gave him the capacity to reason.

To these political theorists, the capacity to reason was the unique domain of the male gender. This followed the same thinking of the ancient Greeks such as Aristotle, who believed that only men have the capacity to transcend their more animalistic needs, while women are best suited to the more primal duties of the home. Rousseau and his contemporaries agreed that women are closer to nature in some ways but saw women as serving a more instrumental purpose for men. Whereas the Greeks saw women as providing the sustenance of life (cooking, cleaning, tending to children) so that men could be freed to debate in the public sphere, Enlightenment thinkers viewed women as offering a civilizing influence for men. Thus, rather than seeing women as simply servants of men, Rousseau tipped his hat to women by suggesting that women are purer and more civilized. Without women to civilize men, chaos would ensue. And though one might conclude that their purity and civility would qualify women for public leadership, Rousseau was able to avoid this logical trap by claiming that breastfeeding is proof that nature intended for women to nurture babies above all. Since nature endowed women with breasts, women must be best suited to domestic life and men to their protection.

Embodied Politics

Rousseau was neither the first nor the only Enlightenment thinker to assign women's political role to familial duties based on the supposed laws of nature. John Locke's *Two Treatises of Government* (1690), published seventy years before Rousseau's *Émile*, introduced a political role for women as part of his rebuttal to those arguing in favour of absolute monarchy (Kerber 1976). Drawing on the story of Adam and Eve, Locke sought to demonstrate that within nature men and women enter a social contract that entitles them to the same rights and responsibilities, although their duties were to be found in separate spheres. Montesquieu (1689–1755) likewise suggested that women would benefit from greater equity in a democratic system than under despotic rule but offered few specifics as to how women could exercise their political power (Kerber 1976).

Despite these hints at the potential for women's agency, it was Rousseau who was most successful at justifying the denial of political rights to women, the poor, and people of colour, by attaching rights to bodies. As Joan Wallach Scott writes,

> There is no denying the presence of bodies – of the physical traits of sex and skin colour – in the political debates of the French Revolution. Whether we take the conflicting opinions expressed during the writing of constitutions, the arguments about slave, mulatto or women's civic rights propounded by Barnave, Brissot, Condorcet or Robespierre, the contrasting reflections of Edmund Burke and Mary Wollstonecraft, or the minutes of section meetings in Paris, we find interpretations that assume that bodies and rights alike could be thought of as "natural" and that this "naturalness" provided a connection between them. Rights were often referred to as being inscribed on bodies, inalienably attached to them, indelibly imprinted on human minds or hearts. But the connection between "natural" bodies and "natural" rights were neither transparent nor straightforward. The meanings of nature, rights, and bodies, as well as the relationships between them, were at issue in the revolutionary debates and these contests about meanings were contests about power. (1989, 1–2)

Numerous revolutionary male leaders drew on the themes most attributed to Rousseau to suggest that women were unsuited to political life because it would lead women to abandon their natural duties to their families. Scott cites Pierre-Gaspard Chaumette, "a radical hébertist and member of the Paris commune" (1989, 3) who rejected women's petition to be included in the radical socialist government; Chaumette stated, "Since

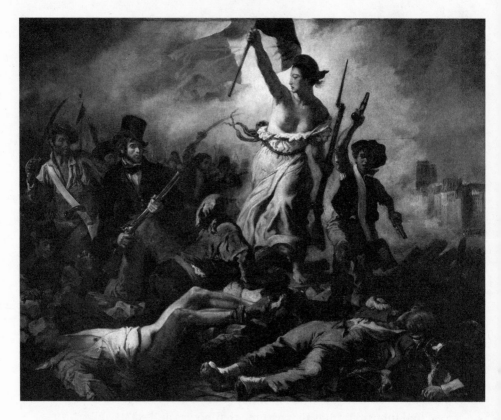

6.1 *La liberté guidant le peuple* (*Liberty Leading the People*), by Eugène Delacroix, 1830.

when is it permitted to give up one's sex? Since when is it decent to see women abandoning the pious cares of their households, the cribs of their children, to come to public places, to harangues in the galleries, at the bar of the senate? Is it to men that nature confided domestic cares? Has she given us breasts to feed our children?" (3)

To these thinkers, breasts are the physical evidence of women's proper allocation to the domestic sphere. Interestingly, at the same time, we also see iconic imagery of breasts as personifying freedom. In *La Liberté guidant le peuple* (*Liberty Leading the People*) by Eugène Delacroix (1830), a bare-chested Marianne leads the people to victory in the French Revolution. As Schiebinger writes, "It is remarkable that in the heady days of the French Revolution, when revolutionaries marched behind the martial and bare-breasted Liberty, the maternal breast became nature's sign that women belonged only in the home" (1993, 408–9). Thus, we see again the long-standing historical pattern of elevating breasts to mythical proportions while simultaneously using their existence to justify women's subordinate status.

Further, breastfeeding served as a powerful rhetorical tool that could bridge political thinking across ideological divides in the eighteenth century, much as it continues to do today. Although Mary Wollstonecraft, the most famous of the eighteenth-century proto-feminists, criticized Rousseau for his claims that women have an inferior capacity for reason, she was in full support of his arguments about breastfeeding. In fact, breastfeeding had become normatively acceptable by the late eighteenth century among the middle and upper classes, particularly because of the pervasive practice of employing wet nurses (Richards 2009; Schiebinger 1993). According to Cynthia Richards, among Wollstonecraft and her husband William Godwin's "radical circle it [maternal nursing] had been firmly embraced" (2009, 567). Richards goes on to explain,

> More importantly, Wollstonecraft herself repeatedly draws her readers' attention to the propriety of such scenes [of nursing], including in the uncompleted *The Wrongs of Woman; or Maria* (1798), a work that Godwin was editing at the same time he was writing *Memoirs*, and which he published simultaneously. In that novel, Wollstonecraft begins with an image of nursing, as she first makes concrete Maria's recent loss of her infant daughter through evoking the pain of her engorged breasts. In her personal letters, Wollstonecraft writes happily, even boastfully, of the pleasure she took in nursing her own daughter, Fanny; and since *The Vindication of the Rights of Woman* (1792), even before her daughter was born, Wollstonecraft has advocated maternal breastfeeding for theoretical reasons. Breastfeeding renders women's bodies capable of active and productive virtue, she argues, and not mere objects of passive display. In *Letters Written during a Short Residence* (1796), this argument becomes the cornerstone of her defence of the much maligned Queen Matilda (a fairly transparent stand-in for Wollstonecraft herself) whose strength of character is borne out through her insistence on suckling her daughter against the wishes of the Danish court. (2009, 568)

Thus, by highlighting the healing powers of women's bodies rather than the dangerous or wicked powers of women, breastfeeding became grounds for women's equality and not only for women's subordination.

Breastfeeding as Civic Duty

Rousseau was greatly assisted in his claim of scientific "proof" of men's and women's natural differences, particularly in his hugely popular book *Émile, or On Education* ([1762] 2011), after Linneaus had formulated his taxonomy of species defining the class *Mammalia* in 1758 (P.A. Weiss 1987; Weiss and Harper 1990). In the book, Rousseau tells the hypothetical story of a young man named *Émile*, who undergoes what Rousseau considered to be the ideal education of an individual. Couched in pseudoscientific claims about anatomy, Rousseau also takes the opportunity to denounce elite mothers as selfish, lazy, and vain, for practices such as swaddling infants or employing a wet nurse. He recounts horrors of wet nurses swaddling infants so tightly that they turn purple in the face or seeing a baby who "is hung on a nail like a sack of clothes, and while the nurse looks after her business, the unfortunate is thus crucified" (Book I, para. 37). These supposed abuses add fuel to Rousseau's argument that the best way to ensure a functioning society is to ensure that mothers breastfeed their own children. As shown in the epigraph to this chapter, not only was it selfish and lazy to fail to breastfeed, in Rousseau's view, but responsibility for all social order was laid on the breasts of mothers. As Schiebinger writes,

> Returning to nature and its laws was seen as the surest way to end corruption and regenerate the state, morally as well as economically. Rousseau, the era's self-appointed spokesman for nature, saw the refusal of mothers to nurse as the source of national depravity. "Everything follows successively from this first depravity. The whole moral order degenerates; naturalness is extinguished in all hearts." The bond between mother and child created through maternal nursing was idealized as the basis of civil society, fostering love of sons for mothers, returning husbands to wives. The infant was imagined to imbibe with breast milk the mother's noble character, her love and virtue. "Let mothers deign to nurse their children," Rousseau preached, "morals will reform themselves, nature's sentiments will be awakened in every heart, the state will be repeopled." (1993, 408)

According to philosopher Rebecca Kukla (2005), it was in large part the theorizing of Rousseau that shifted dominant dichotomies from good and bad woman (saint versus witch) to good and bad mother, whom she calls the "Fetish Mother" (how we are supposed to be) and the "Unruly Mother" (what we are to avoid being). She draws on Marx's use of the term "fetish" to describe objects "perceived as having inherent normative value and power" (82). She explains,

My claim is that the "natural" maternal body, and especially the body of the nursing mother, can be productively interpreted as functioning as a social fetish in Post-Revolutionary Western culture – that is, it is experienced as an inherent, atomic source of social (as opposed to economic, sexual, or divine) value and power. Her body is a perfect and uninterrupted whole, which includes the body of her fetus or infant. The Fetish Mother enjoys an uninterrupted "natural" unity with her child. The space of her body includes her infant, which begins inside of her and is then sutured to her naturally through her breast and its milk. The surface of her body is a public spectacle symbolizing the possibility of well-ordered human nature free from hysterical incoherence, artificial hybrids, or deformed monstrosity. (82)

Thus, drawing on appeals to nature as grounds for moral decision-making, the breastfeeding mother becomes identified as the moral ideal upon which social order depends.

In contrast to the Fetish Mother is the Unruly Mother, who, like the witches before her, is defined by her lack of order and her unpredictability. As Kukla goes on to write,

the Unruly Mother is a volatile, fragile, contingent, appetitive being, with little resistance against temptation, craving, and the extremities of passion. She is governed not by orderly principles but by an ad hoc, capricious logic of sentiment and craving. Easily penetrated, she must be carefully regulated, policed, and controlled, for her disorderly nature is always at risk of hysteria, and this hysteria is highly contagious – it will deform her offspring and through them transmit itself to the body politic. Her powers are no less than those of the Fetish Mother, but she cannot be trusted to carry out her enormous social and moral responsibilities without oversight and governance. The spaces of her body and home must be relocated to the public domain and rendered panoptic so as to make them manageable by responsible, more stable social and scientific institutions. Through such public discipline and surveillance, the Unruly Mother will hopefully be prevented from inappropriately ingesting things, leaking things, and unnaturally disordering and separating that which ought to remain harmonized and unified. (2005, 83–4)

Kukla's argument also points to a contradiction between, on the one hand, the idealization of breasts of symbols of liberty and, on the other hand, the suspicion that women need to have their bodies controlled because they can't be trusted to step outside of their allocated domestic sphere. Rousseau might not have been so desperate to protect society through the promotion of breastfeeding had it not been for the changing economic conditions that led to the rise of wet-nursing during the eighteenth century.

Although wet-nursing has been critiqued since at least Aristotle (Papastavrou et al. 2015), the eighteenth century saw a huge rise in both the practice and its critiques. With the development of factories, mothers could not take their infants to work and therefore needed milk substitutes to feed their infants. For free but poor women, wet-nursing became a thriving career option (Hufton 1975; Sussman 1977). According to Schiebinger (1993), up to 90 per cent of children in Paris and Lyon went to wet nurses by the 1780s. Social concern regarding the rise in wet-nursing was not only for the babies but also for society as a whole. Schiebinger explains, "Fears began to grow that Europe's population was declining at a time when governments were looking for increased labor power to bolster military and economic expansion. The concern to increase population was so great in Denmark, for example, that a law was passed in 1707 authorizing young women to bear as many children as possible even if they were bastards" (405).

Although men had historically denigrated breastfeeding, the Enlightenment brought a generation of men who denigrated women for *not* breastfeeding. In some ways the exhortations against wet-nursing were founded in a genuine health concern. According to historian George Sussman's (1977) analysis of the limited available data on wet-nursing in eighteenth- and nineteenth-century France, of the 1,653 registered infants placed with wet nurses in four rural arrondissements from 1814 to 1825, 26.5 percent died. According to Schiebinger, "Linnaeus – himself a practicing physician – prepared a dissertation against the evils of wet-nursing in 1752 just a few years before coining the term *Mammalia* and while watching his own children suckle." Linnaeus saw wet-nursing as a violation of natural laws that would harm mothers and babies by denying infants colostrum, which he claimed was "crucial for purging the child of meconium," but also "most nurses came from the poorest classes, they ate fatty foods, drank too much alcohol, were riddled with pox and venereal disease – all of which produced unhealthy, if not lethal milk" (Schiebinger 1993, 405).

Those concerned about the dangers of wet-nursing, including Linnaeus, Rousseau, and British physician William Cadogan, often framed their pleas to end the practice by focusing on the character defects of mothers who did not breastfeed their own children, such as by alleging that women didn't breastfeed out of vanity, or that they lied about their reasons for not breastfeeding. For example, "Linnaeus charged that women only pretended to be unable to breast-feed and ridiculed their many 'excuses': that they did not have enough milk, or could not be deprived of fluids precious to their own health, or were overloaded with domestic affairs" (Schiebinger 1993, 408). Both Linnaeus and Rousseau suggested that not breastfeeding had something to do with women wanting to have sex with their husbands or not wanting to have sex with their husbands, respectively. Neither attitude toward sex with one's husband was viewed positively (Schiebinger 1993).

These ideas have stuck around ever since. According to Kukla, the language used by these eighteenth-century men does not differ much from the language used to describe the importance of breastfeeding today:

> The Rousseauian imagination has persisted, with anthropologist Ashley Montague declaring in 1971 that the "breastfeeding relationship constitutes the foundation for the development of all human relationships" (Montagu 1971, 77) and, very recently, the American Academy of Pediatrics opening their policy statement on breastfeeding by extolling the "benefits of breastfeeding to the infant, the mother and the nation." (Kukla 2005, 159)

We can further see this in calls to breastfeed in order to save governments money, such as in a recent "news" story with the headline "Lack of breastfeeding costs global economy nearly $1B every day" (Yi 2019). Without diving into a critique of these contemporary examples, suffice it to say that the idea that breastfeeding is a civic duty remains persuasive to many.

Women's Resistance and the *Querelle des femmes*

Though macrostructural shifts including demographic changes, rising infant mortality, revolutionary thinking, and the introduction of science and its attendant death of God offer clues as to why breastfeeding became a central concern for Enlightenment thinkers, I offer another possible hypothesis for why these men were so fixated on breastfeeding as evidence for women's natural duties. If their goal was purely to preserve the superior status of men, they could have chosen any number of other ways to identify women's inferiority. Many religions have suggested that menstruation is unclean, for example, and the ancient Greeks suggested that women's wombs wander, making women "crazy." Though infants were dying with wet nurses, one could have suggested alternative reforms to address mothers' and wet nurses' needs – or larger approaches to address widespread poverty. If the issue was simply infant feeding, why the need to moralize women's bodies more generally?

I would argue that at least some of the concern these men felt about breastfeeding had much to do with winning a rhetorical battle of the sexes, known as the *querelle des femmes*. Although the term "feminism" did not exist until the nineteenth century (Hicks 2015) and most discussions of feminist movements consider the "first wave" to have occurred in the late nineteenth and early twentieth centuries, according to historian Joan Kelly (1982), there was a four-hundred-year-old tradition of women thinking about gender politics in Europe that predates the French Revolution. Though powerful elites had effectively stunted the collective capacity of peasant women to overthrow the ruling structures, there remained women with greater privilege who were able to use their social and economic status to insulate themselves from the personal risks that came with challenging dominant patriarchal orthodoxy. As Eileen Hunt Botting writes,

> The *querelle des femmes*, or intellectual debate on women, had flourished in French, Italian, and English courts, salons, and convents since Christine de Pisan published *The Book of the City of Ladies* in 1405. Descartes's theory of the mind as separate from the body had led generations of French feminist thinkers – most famously, seventeenth-century philosopher Francois Poulain de la Barre – to claim the mind (and hence morality) has no sex. (2017, 739)

Unlike later feminists, these women tended to focus their efforts only on the written word, without any calls for collective action or a wider feminist movement. However, their intellectual claim that women were men's intellectual equals was quite radical for the time (Kelly 1982).

In addition to de Pisan (Italy, 1364–1430), other women engaged in the *querelle* included Lucrezia Marinella (Italy, 1571–1653), Rachel Speght (England, 1597–unknown), Bathsua Makin (England, 1600–75), Aphra Behn (England, 1640–89), Mary Astell (England, 1666–1731), Judith Drake (England, 1670s–1723), and Elizabeth Elstob (England, 1683–1756), all of whom were married to or the daughters of well-educated and/or economically successful men. You might think of them as the original White liberal feminists, a kind of cadre of early Betty Friedans. These White bourgeois women had the privilege of attaining some private education but were denied access to formal educational institutions. Thus, their reading in the modern humanities gave them a consciousness about the possibilities of individual liberty and agency, while the patriarchal social structure frustrated their desires to be treated as true equals. Kelly explains, "In the main, the early feminist theorists were the forebears of what Virginia Woolf called 'the daughters of educated men' – daughters in revolt against the fathers who schooled some of them for a society they forbade all women to enter" (1982, 8).

Sitting in a position of relative privilege meant these highly educated women had the time and the means to pull no punches in their critiques of male dominance, often in the form of short pamphlets. These women refused to go gently into submission and were brutal in their often funny critiques of the apparent shortcomings of the male mind. However, unlike their male adversaries who actively attacked women by citing Scripture or words of other misogynists, these proto-feminists relied on careful critical analyses of text and logic over appeals to authority:

> Every learned tradition was subject to feminist critique, since all
> were dominated by men and justified male subjection of women.
> Feminist wit penetrated to the core of male pretension in the
> irrefutable arguments and commonsensical adages that supported
> men's power over women. Strength of mind certainly goes along
> with strength of body, Mary Astell concurred; "and 'tis only for some
> odd accidents, which philosophers have not yet thought worthwhile

to enquire into, that the sturdiest porter is not the wisest man."
Aristotelians were held up to ridicule for their phallic conception of
woman as a mutilated and/or impotent male. If women appeared as
"imperfect men" to Aristotle, doubtless that was because "they are
deficient in that ornament of the chin, a beard – what else [could
he mean]?" But deeper than wit, the feminists saw that the learning
they inherited was not merely biased, it was deeply flawed by male
interest in maintaining the supremacy of men ... The women noted
that male authors appealed to nature and reason to "explain" the ex-
clusion of women from learning, government, and public office, but
we "ought to have better proofs ... than the bare word of the persons
who advance [such arguments], as their being parties so immediately
concerned must render all they say of this kind highly suspicious."
(Kelly 1982, 19–20)

Rather than arguing that their opponents were being unfair, unjust,
or immoral, these early feminists were attacking them on the grounds of
bias, poor logic, and insufficient evidence for their claims. One common
way that these women would poke holes in sexist premises was by referring to "women worthies": "historical or contemporary women conspicu-
ous for their merit" (Hicks 2015, 175). They might point to Joan of Arc or
the Amazons to challenge the claim that women are incapable of military
might or cite Sappho's brilliance to dispute women's intellectual inferiority. Although some later feminists, especially Mary Wollstonecraft, have
dismissed the value of indexing uniquely impressive women, many of
those engaged in the *querelle* found this to be an effective strategy in their
argumentation.

One highly popular proto-feminist pamphlet during "an outbreak of the
querelle des femmes in 1739" (Hicks 2015, 177) was authored by "Sophia," the
name given as author of an otherwise anonymous series of pamphlets, attributed either to Lady Mary Wortley Montague (1689–1762) or to Lady
Sophia Fermor (1724–45). Interestingly, the name Sophia is of Greek deriv-
ation and means "wisdom." These tracts, titled *Woman Not Inferior to Man*
(Sophia 1739) and *Woman's Superior Excellence over Man* (Sophia 1740), were
a response to yet another insult to women's intelligence published in an
article in the serial *Common Sense*. According to Philip Hicks, "Not content with mere equality with men, Sophia made a bid for superiority over
them, claiming transcendent beauty, eloquence, and virtue for her sex. She

also insisted upon women's fitness for the offices of military general, privy councillor, judge, and professor" (2015, 178).

Reading Sophia's *Woman not Inferior to Man: Or, a Short and Modest Vindication of the Natural Right of the Fair-Sex to a Perfect Equality of Power, Dignity, and Esteem with the Men* led me to actually laugh out loud in a number of places and fill the comment boxes of my PDF with lots of exclamation marks at her gutsy writing. She ridicules male philosophers and asserts that using reason to claim that women are inferior is to impose silence on them. She refers to the ancient ruler Cato as a fool and an exemplar of "half-thinking retailers of sentences" and states that the "sages" and "divine oracles" of old are "as oafish as the dupes who revere them" (1739, chap. 4, paras. 4–5).

However, Sophia (1739) did not simply insult male thinkers and their followers but carefully framed a dialectical response to the ideas being batted around in the *querelle*. In the main she was arguing against the overlapping claims of the day that (1) women are on earth for men's use, (2) women cannot govern, lead armies, serve as clergy, be educated, or teach in universities, and (3) women's purpose on earth is to "breed and nurse children" (chap. 2, para. 1) because (a) men are physically stronger than women, (b) men have a greater capacity to reason and think, (c) women are too emotional, and (d) educating women would make them "proud and vicious" (chap. 3, para. 8). Sadly, she failed to put these arguments to bed, considering that I have heard them all used in my lifetime, but she nonetheless offered an extremely persuasive critique of these claims that would likely have even the most pro-feminist man feeling ill at ease.

Notably, she begins her critique by noting that breastfeeding is "held by the *Men* in a despicable light, as something low and degrading" (Sophia 1739, chap. 2, para. 2). In contrast to the later male philosophers who suggested that women are too vain, lazy, or selfish to breastfeed, Sophia points the finger at men for discouraging women from the practice. Although she begins her treatise by challenging this degradation of breastfeeding, she is merely descriptive, not prescriptive; in other words, she is not trying to suggest that women *should* breastfeed, just that they do. However, she argues that because women breastfeed, they should be valued above men because breastfeeding has allowed humans to exist, making it a more essential occupation than any other across time or culture. She challenges the notion of the higher valuing of soldiers or statesmen, since they are neither found nor necessary in a state of nature, whereas the need for breastfeeding is universal. She further suggests that given women's capacity to breastfeed, men are also dependent on women, at least as much as women are dependent on men. Not only do women nurse men as babies, but for men to gain esteem through their children they depend on women to raise and nurture them.

According to Sophia, men have two possible means by which to control women: with reason or with their violent "passions" that put women "upon the level with brutes" (1739, chap. 2, paras. 8, 7). If reason is employed, then women must have the capacity to understand logic and reasoning, which would mean that they are above brute animals. Further, if both men and women have the capacity to reason, and men are truly committed to the use of reason to justify their behaviour, then

> No matter by what mouth *reason* speaks: if *Men* were strictly attach'd to it; whether we or themselves were the vehicles of its influence, we shou'd on both sides be equally determin'd by it. But the case is at present quite otherwise. The *Men* who cannot deny us to be rational creatures, wou'd have us justify their irrational opinion and treatment of us, by descending to a mean compliance with their irrational Expectations. (1739, chap. 2, para. 9)

Given that men use violence rather than reason to assert their dominance, men are the truly vain and emotionally needy, indicating a lesser capacity to govern than women. She concludes her summary by applying deductive logic to the Cartesian belief that the body and soul are separate, as follows: Given that sex differences are found only in the body, not the soul; that body sex differences relate only to reproduction, that is, men's and women's brains are the same and "we hear with ears, see with eyes, and taste with a tongue as well as they" (Sophia 1739, chap. 3, para. 8); that God connects the souls of women and men to their respective bodies; and that this union of body and soul is cemented by "sentiments, passions, and propensions" (para. 5); then we can conclude that all diversity comes from "*education, exercise,* and the *impressions* of those external objects which surround us in different Circumstances" (para. 4). In other words, differences in men's and women's heretofore demonstrated capacities have been a result of nurture, not nature.

Given this logic, Sophia suggests then that all the ills attributed to women are a result of their lack of education. Further, their mistreatment has been a result of men's jealousy of women's greater gifts, including breastfeeding. Thus, she sets out to articulate further why women should be educated on an even level with men and why women are better suited than men for most forms of public office. Though men claim that women can govern neither themselves nor others, Sophia suggests any shortcomings women may have at self-governance can be explained by men's "circumvention, treachery, and baseness." She goes on to note that women have been robbed of their natural right to education that would have taught them how to govern, but men have no such excuse. Considering that "they have all the advantages requisite to qualify them; and, if, spite of all, we are worse under their government than under our own; the consequence speaks itself, that either they have a natural want of capacity, or want of honesty" (1739, chap. 4, para. 1).

She goes on to suggest that women would also make better professors than men because of women's "loquacity" (Sophia 1739, chap. 6, para. 1) and ability to speak fluidly and freely, compared to men's awkwardness with public speaking. As she writes,

> With what hesitation, confusion, and drudgery, do not the *Men* labour to bring forth their thoughts? And when they do utter something tolerable, with what insipid gestures, distortions, and grimaces, do they murder the few good things they say? Whereas, when a *Woman* speaks, her air is generally noble and preventing, her gesture free, and full of dignity, her action is decent, her words are easy and insinuating, her stile [*sic*] is pathetic and winning, and her voice melodious, and tuned to her subject. She can soar to a level with the highest intellect without bombast, and with a complacency natural to the delicacy of her frame, descend to the meanest capacity without meanness. (Sophia 1739, chap. 6, para. 2)

Though one can note a slight flaw in her logic that women's weaknesses are a result of their education but their gifts come from their nature, we could also interpret this as her simply throwing shade or implying that if women's nature is a certain way, according to men, then just imagine how much better women would be within an environment that nurtured their potential as well. She likely intended this latter idea, as she uses this logic to suggest that women's natural eloquence makes for better judges, magistrates, lawyers, ministers, and teachers. She also gets in a dig at philosophers who waste time on the "*Entia Rationis*, fictious trifles, no where to be found but in their own noddles" (or their noodles, for the American or Canadian reader) (Sophia 1739, chap. 6, para. 5).

Sophia (1739) suggests that women would do philosophy or theology differently than men, because women would focus on more practical matters with greater humility than do men. Thus, she notes that if women were to "express our conceptions of God, it wou'd never enter into the head of any one of us to describe him as a venerable old man. No, we have a more noble idea of him, than to compare him to any thing created" (chap. 6, para. 6). To her, God may have intentionally forbidden women from becoming religious leaders because men were in greater need of religious teachings, owing to "the general tendency of the *Men* to *impiety* and *irreligion*" (chap. 6, para. 9).

After going on to explain why women are also better suited than men to lead armies, Sophia concludes by dialling back her claims, reassuring the reader that she is not trying to foment a revolution against men or to

> invert the present order of things, with regard to *government* and
> *authority*. No, let them stand as they are: I only mean to shew my sex,
> that they are not so despicable as the *Men* wou'd have them believe
> themselves, and that we are capable of as much greatness of soul
> as the best of that haughty sex. And I am fully convinced, it wou'd
> be to the joint interest of both to think so. (1739, chap. 8, para. 1)

She concludes her work by encouraging women to "throw aside idle amusements, and to betake themselves to the improvement of their minds, that we may be able to act with that becoming dignity our nature has fitted us to" (1739, chap. 8, para. 7). Her hope is that, by educating themselves, women will be able to garner enough respect to show men that they deserve better treatment.

Though by today's standards Sophia's goal is a modest one, I can imagine that male readers of the day would have been rather perturbed by the arguments. Not only does she insult men's intelligence, but she has the audacity to suggest that women are better suited to nearly all pursuits and that men are as useless as extra lumber on a ship (her metaphor, not mine). Despite her statements to the contrary, her concluding argument that it would be in both men's and women's interests to recognize that women have equal capacity to men could be taken as a veiled threat of male overthrow.

This fear may have been particularly acute given that Sophia's writings were hugely popular (Hicks 2015) and sparked widespread debate across Europe. According to Göller, the publication of the Sophia pamphlets was a revolutionary landmark in the progress of feminist movement, offering "practically a compendium of all the arguments and counter-arguments advanced since the Restoration on the upbringing and education of the fair sex" (1983, 84). All three of Sophia's treatises were reprinted together in 1751, which, Edith Kuiper notes, was a time in which "feminist challenges to male hegemony began thus to bubble up through an increasing number of fissures" (2006, 43). It also coincided with the creation of the "Bluestockings": women dedicated to the education of women who met in groups to discuss and write about women's advancement (Bodek 1976). Like the women of the *querelle*, the Bluestockings remained more focused on writing than actively protesting; nonetheless, they challenged the separation of public and private spheres for the harm they cause by blocking women from their full potential (Kuiper 2006).

Jean-Jacques Gives Birth to *Émile*

Given that this rising tide of proto-feminism coincided with the revolutionary fervour that sought to overthrow the French and British monarchies, we can see why European men might have felt threatened at the prospect of an impending gender revolution. Although I have yet to find a historian or a philosopher making this case, I read *Émile* as a direct response to Sophia. Put another way, *Émile* is not Rousseau's thesis but rather an anti-thesis, used to stanch the potential power of Sophia's words and logic. This would answer the puzzling question of *why* Rousseau felt compelled to situate breastfeeding not only as central to women's essential nature but also as their responsibility and civic duty. Further, this makes sense given that Rousseau began his philosophy career as an assistant to Madame Dupin, an important philosopher of the period known for her writings on gender equity. Such an assignment would have deeply immersed him in eighteenth-century French egalitarian feminist thought, as documented by political scientist Eileen Hunt Botting (2017). In fact, Botting argues that early Rousseau followed the arguments developed by Madame Dupin that gender inequality was a social construction:

> We can better situate his early writings on women in the context of his secretariat to Madame Dupin from 1745 to 1751 as well as broader

trends in the French Enlightenment's intervention in the *querelle des femmes* – or the intellectual debate on the capabilities of women in comparison to men that had raged in Europe and its colonies since the early 1400s. Secondly, understanding the composition of the "Critique" as a complex collaboration among several persons, including Madame Dupin and Rousseau, leads us to see how the early Rousseau robustly converged in feminist ideas with one of the great woman philosophers of the age, before he gradually diverged from this egalitarian school of thought over the course of the 1750s to develop the full-fledged patriarchal political theory for which he is famous. (733–4)

However, Botting (2017) does not explain how and why Rousseau transformed from an early advocate for feminist arguments into a guiding voice for the maintenance of a patriarchal status quo. Rousseau's own writing may contain the answer. In the preface to *Émile*, he wrote,

This collection of scattered thoughts and observations has little order or continuity; it was begun to give pleasure to a good mother who thinks for herself. My first idea was to write a tract a few pages long, but I was carried away by my subject, and before I knew what I was doing my tract had become a kind of book, too large indeed for the matter contained in it, but too small for the subject of which it treats. For a long time I hesitated whether to publish it or not, and I have often felt, when at work upon it, that it is one thing to publish a few pamphlets and another to write a book. (Rousseau [1762] 2011, author's preface, para. 1)

Thus, we see our first clues that he is responding to an unnamed "good mother" in writing this work that began as a series of ideas to be published in pamphlets. He also seems rather keen on humbling himself throughout the work, perhaps to defend against the accusations Sophia had lodged against the men engaged in the *querelle*, describing them as haughty and vain and in need of great flattery. For example, Rousseau writes,

When I freely express my opinion, I have so little idea of claiming authority that I always give my reasons, so that you may weigh and judge them for yourselves; but though I would not obstinately defend my ideas, I think it my duty to put them forward; for the principles with regard to which I differ from other writers are not matters of indifference; we must know whether they are true or false, for on them depends the happiness or the misery of mankind. (author's preface, para. 5)

He also seems to be defending himself against Sophia's critique of male philosophers who rely on appeals to authority over reason, fail to ground their theories in empirical evidence, and focus on nothing of practical utility, when he emphatically states,

People are always telling me to make PRACTICABLE suggestions. You might as well tell me to suggest what people are doing already, or at least to suggest improvements which may be incorporated with the wrong methods at present in use. There are matters with regard to which such a suggestion is far more chimerical than my own, for in such a connection the good is corrupted and the bad is none the better for it. I would rather follow exactly the established method than adopt a better method by halves. There would be fewer contradictions in the man; he cannot aim at one and the same time at two different objects. Fathers and mothers, what you desire that you can do. May I count on your goodwill? (author's preface, para. 5)

Rousseau seems to be speaking directly to Sophia's critique that women would do philosophy better than men, being more focused on practical and important matters compared with the chimerical whims of men. Thus, he refutes the claim that he is full of himself but also maintains that new methods are not likely to be useful.

Not only do Rousseau's words and the tone he seeks to set in the preface accord with Sophia's critique, but so does the entire purpose of the work and its arguments. *Émile* is a treatise on how education should be carried out rather than a critique of how education is carried out, and thereby it sidesteps Sophia's suggestion that women should be allowed to enter the hallowed halls of the educational system *as it stands*. Additionally, by framing his arguments around a moral call to the ideal society, as Penny Weiss (1987) cogently argues, rather than focusing directly on men's and women's different capacities, Rousseau quashes the claim that women should be allowed full participation on the basis that they are already naturally equal, although distinct. In other words, unlike many men before him, Rousseau allows that women are just as naturally capable as men – but twists Sophia's claim to women's moral superiority to show that there is a benefit to society if we create a new educational system that values women while maintaining clear differences in men's and women's social roles.

Specifically, Rousseau outlines the key sex differences in terms of physical strength, mental capacities, reproduction, and interests and disposition. Notably, these are the same key points made by Sophia. Weiss (1987) points out the multitude of ways in which Rousseau uses terms like "ought" rather than "are" to show that these differences are beneficial to society, even if they are not part of women's nature. Thus, for example, Rousseau sees civilized culture as what causes women to be weaker, not that women's weakness makes them more civilized or socially marginalized. He sees a social benefit in women cultivating their weakness to ensure that men feel useful and to motivate men to engage in socially important tasks they might otherwise shirk. This would thus offer a counter-argument against those, like Sophia, who suggest that men are so useless as to be used only as our bulwarks in battle.

Rousseau agrees that women have the capacity to reason and refutes Aristotle's suggestion that women are as base as animals, ordained by God to be ruled by men. As Weiss writes,

> It is important to remember that in Rousseau's state of nature, human rationality is hardly distinguishable from that of other animals. In this sense, any development of intellectual capacities is unnatural, and must be accounted for primarily by environmental (including educational) influences. Also, like many other capacities to evolve only under certain contingent circumstances, Rousseau does not consider the awakening of rationality to be wholly unproblematic and good in its social or personal consequences ... Intellectual achievement per se offers no guarantee of personal or social well-being. Education of the intellect can and should be manipulated and constrained by factors that have but little to do with the innate capacities of the sexes. (1987, 87)

Thus, if Sophia's contention is that women should be allowed to be educated because they are at least as capable as men, Rousseau cleverly can allow for her to be right about women's capabilities while challenging her assumption on the benefits of education itself. Thus, as Weiss (1987) explains, Rousseau is no biological determinist but more of a structural functionalist, who sees that a society will be best ordered if men and women have distinct roles. Even in his discussion of reproduction, he draws little on biological differences in men's and women's natures. In fact, "Women have no 'maternal instinct' in Rousseau's thought, as that concept is usually understood. In the state of nature, women nurse children to relieve themselves of milk, and perhaps respond to a child's cries out of pity, a sentiment common to both sexes. Beyond that, any attachment to children arises from the habit of living with them, and to this men are equally susceptible" (90). Rousseau thus encourages domesticity for women not because they are *naturally* better at it but as a means to engineer a better and happier social order than one would even find in the state of nature (P.A. Weiss 1987). By comparing this quote to Sophia's work, we can also see that Rousseau's dismissal of breastfeeding as simply something women did to relieve their own physical discomfort in a state of nature denies the value that Sophia suggests breastfeeding grants women.

Nonetheless, we know that Rousseau saw breastfeeding as the key to bringing about a moral order, as described in this chapter's epigraph. In fact, as he writes in a footnote, "The earliest education is most important and it undoubtedly is woman's work. If the author of nature had meant to assign it to men he would have given them milk to feed the child." ([1762] 2011, Book 1, para. 2). However, Rousseau admits that men and women have an equivalent natural capacity to nurture children. He also concedes that there are some women who are stronger than some men and that women's greater concern for what people think of them is a result of environmental differences in their upbringing, not differences in interest or disposition. And in a rather sly use of logic that seems almost like a direct shot at Sophia in particular, he even notes that Cato, the ancient ruler Sophia derides in *Woman Not Inferior to Man*, was a highly involved father:

When we read in Plutarch that Cato the Censor, who ruled Rome with such glory, brought up his own sons from the cradle, and so carefully that he left everything to be present when their nurse, that is to say their mother, bathed them; when we read in Suetonius that Augustus, the master of the world which he had conquered and which he himself governed, himself taught his grandsons to write, to swim, to understand the beginnings of science, and that he always

had them with him, we cannot help smiling at the little people of
those days who amused themselves with such follies, and who were
too ignorant, no doubt, to attend to the great affairs of the great
people of our own time. (Book I, para. 60)

Fundamentally, *Émile* appears to build off Sophia's arguments while
twisting them to men's advantage. Yes, women's weaknesses are a result of
their education, Rousseau is saying, but then so too are men's. He writes,

God makes all things good; man meddles with them and they
become evil. He forces one soil to yield the products of another,
one tree to bear another's fruit. He confuses and confounds time,
place, and natural conditions. He mutilates his dog, his horse, and
his slave. He destroys and defaces all things; he loves all that is
deformed and monstrous; he will have nothing as nature made it,
not even man himself, who must learn his paces like a saddle-horse,
and be shaped to his master's taste like the trees in his garden. Yet
things would be worse without this education, and mankind cannot
be made by halves. Under existing conditions a man left to himself
from birth would be more of a monster than the rest. Prejudice,
authority, necessity, example, all the social conditions into which we
are plunged, would stifle nature in him and put nothing in her place.
(Book I, para. 1)

Given the distortion of men's true nature by misguided human med-
dling, he argues that we need an entirely new system of education to teach
men how to live in accordance with their natural design. He goes on to
write, "Tender, anxious mother, I appeal to you. You can remove this young
tree from the highway and shield it from the crushing force of social conventions. Tend and water it ere it dies. One day its fruit will reward your
care. From the outset raise a wall round your child's soul; another may
sketch the plan, you alone should carry it into execution" (Book I, para. 2).

It is here that we find the aforementioned notion that children must be
first educated by women given their lactational capacities. However, Rousseau does not simply suggest that mothers should do this and be happy
about it; rather, he acknowledges the sacrifices this demands of mothers and affirms that mothers who nurse their children merit the highest

respect of all, but most especially from their own children. He notes that "if a child could be so unnatural as to fail in respect for the mother who bore him and nursed him at her breast, who for so many years devoted herself to his care, such a monstrous wretch should be smothered at once as unworthy to live" (Book I, para. 2). Here we see the genius of Rousseau. Sophia took for granted that the nursing of children by women is essential to the maintenance of the human race and chastised men for not giving women their due. Rousseau concedes this point but then turns the logic on its head by noting that if nursing is so important, then any failings of men must be the result of maternal failure. He develops his argument based on a nearly obsessive preoccupation with what he considers the dangers of swaddling, resulting from mothers' dereliction of breastfeeding duty:

> Since mothers have despised their first duty and refused to nurse their own children, they have had to be entrusted to hired nurses. Finding themselves the mothers of a stranger's children, without the ties of nature, they have merely tried to save themselves trouble. A child unswaddled would need constant watching; well swaddled it is cast into a corner and its cries are unheeded. So long as the nurse's negligence escapes notice, so long as the nursling does not break its arms or legs, what matter if it dies or becomes a weakling for life. Its limbs are kept safe at the expense of its body, and if anything goes wrong it is not the nurse's fault.
>
> These gentle mothers, having got rid of their babies, devote themselves gaily to the pleasures of the town. Do they know how their children are being treated in the villages? If the nurse is at all busy, the child is hung up on a nail like a bundle of clothes and is left crucified while the nurse goes leisurely about her business. Children have been found in this position purple in the face, their tightly bandaged chest forbade the circulation of the blood, and it went to the head; so the sufferer was considered very quiet because he had not strength to cry. How long a child might survive under such conditions I do not know, but it could not be long. That, I fancy, is one of the chief advantages of swaddling clothes ...
>
> Not content with having ceased to suckle their children, women no longer wish to do it; with the natural result motherhood becomes a burden; means are found to avoid it. They will destroy their work

to begin it over again, and they thus turn to the injury of the race the charm which was given them for its increase. This practice, with other causes of depopulation, forbodes the coming fate of Europe. Her arts and sciences, her philosophy and morals, will shortly reduce her to a desert. She will be the home of wild beasts, and her inhabitants will hardly have changed for the worse. (Book 1, paras. 36–9)

In this rather remarkable slide down a slippery slope of a logical fallacy, Rousseau takes us from a start of life without maternal nursing to the depopulation of Europe, reduced to a desert of wild beasts. To help us avoid the total annihilation of European culture, he offers his modest suggestions in the rest of the book for a better educational system, in which he carefully addresses each claim made by (though unattributed to) Sophia through the case of his hypothetical pupil, *Émile*.

And, as if he really wanted to stick it to her, in the final chapter he names *Émile's* prized wife Sophie – the French form of the name Sophia. We see that Rousseau is responding to broad arguments of the *querelle* but riding on the backs of better thinkers, twisting their arguments to assert his superiority. As my wise sister and first book editor Rosalie Rippey pointed out after reading a draft of this chapter, it's almost as though Rousseau is the original men's rights activist – learning from feminist critiques of gender and then weaponizing them against women.

Mary Wollstonecraft's Puppies

I have no idea how Sophia reacted to Rousseau's treatise, since we do not even know who Sophia was, but the wild popularity of *Émile* has been shown to have contributed to a greater normalization of breastfeeding and social disapproval of wet-nursing among both men and women (Kukla 2005; Schiebinger 1993). Whereas other attacks on women in the *querelle* were roundly disputed by women, no man or woman was going to dispute the benefits of breastfeeding. Thus, by rhetorically situating breastfeeding as central to our species and as a God-given natural gift that can socialize and civilize nations, Rousseau created an argument that feminists struggle to make sense of to this day. In fact, as discussed above, in full agreement with Rousseau's view of breastfeeding was his intellectual admirer and major critic, Mary Wollstonecraft.

Through a cruel twist of fate, however, her love and respect for breast-feeding made the scene of her death both ironic and obscene (Richards 2009). As Wollstonecraft lay dying from puerperal fever – a result of the placenta not being fully delivered after the birth of her second child, the future author Mary Shelley – puppies were placed on her breasts to draw out the milk that was deemed too dangerous for her newborn baby. The ordering of puppies was a somewhat common practice at the time, according to Cynthia Richards (2009), as colostrum was then falsely believed to be dangerous to or at least indigestible by babies. Attaching puppies to the breasts would allow the milk to come in more quickly and prevent pain from engorgement or potential mastitis. Penicillin was yet to be invented, and the failure to properly deliver the placenta, clogged milk ducts, or even the nip of a puppy could lead to a fatal infection.

As told by Wollstonecraft's husband, William Godwin, these actions, however, went against what Wollstonecraft stood for. Citing Jacques Gelis, Richards explains,

> Wollstonecraft's attending doctor "forb[idding] the child's having
> the breast" suggests the milk would be too contaminated to nourish
> the young infant, requiring the doctor to ban the breast ([Gelis 1991,]
> 136). In a broader sense, this view suggests a troubling inversion of
> Wollstonecraft's advocacy of breastfeeding: this "natural" labour
> of the female body turns against both mother and child, in effect
> poisoning them. Those who witnessed death by puerperal fever
> describe the "sickness" as having a "shape of horror and an outward
> monstrosity" [Gelis 1991], and this image of Wollstonecraft suckling
> puppies would seem to act against her best efforts to universalize
> this practice, to render it a normative activity. In this context, Woll-
> stonecraft must breastfeed because her body acts abnormally, and
> the introduction of the puppies only emphasizes the conventional
> view of how dangerous the female body could prove to be. For her
> own protection, Wollstonecraft's daughter is denied the breast, and
> Wollstonecraft must submit to the suckling puppies in order to con-
> tain the monstrous processes of her own body. (2009, 570)

Richards goes on to argue that what made this scene so obscene was actually not the puppies but the fact that Wollstonecraft's milk had been framed as corrupted. This went against all of her Enlightenment ideals, particularly within the context of revolutionary France. Richards cites Mary Jacobus (1992) in explaining that

> the "incorruptible milk" of the Republican mother functioned figuratively in the French Revolution to "purify" both the wrongs of the *ancien régime* and the "disorders" of the Revolution. It united all men within the fraternity and equality of the New Republic, a concept made concrete through the construction of the Fountain of Regeneration on the site of the Bastille and its commemoration in a coin depicting the President of the Convention and representatives "drinking the regenerative waters springing from the breasts of an Egyptian deity." The excess of milk identified medically as a likely source of Wollstonecraft's bodily malfunction does not therefore represent a violation of the Republican order, but rather its affirmation: Wollstonecraft would have plenty for all. Rather, it is the banning of the breast that proves obscene; Wollstonecraft's milk is not incorruptible, but corrupted, with the arrival of the puppies signalling the failure of the mother's milk to serve as a purifying agent and a unifying bond among men. Once again, the normative human behavior, or the "natural" work of the female body, is rendered unnatural in this scene, parodying Wollstonecraft's own ideals and those of her period. (572–3)

Not only did the labelling of her milk as diseased violate the premise of the day that maternal milk was a healing salve for all society, but it also restores the earlier images of women as bestial in comparison with men's greater rationality. As Richards writes, "this image of the suckling puppies seems to affirm this association with the sensual and to conjoin her quite literally with the animalistic." In so doing, it then potentially undermines "Wollstonecraft's efforts to make women's full enfranchisement essential towards human progress" (2009, 572). Maternal breastfeeding becomes no act of virtue or evidence of women's capacity to transcend their animal natures but is rather little different than a dog nursing her pups.

The tale of Mary Wollstonecraft's death illuminates the limitations of defining the value of a gender by a single bodily function. When women's natural work of breastfeeding fails to function properly, what is the value of a woman's life to become? The story also reaffirms that the connection

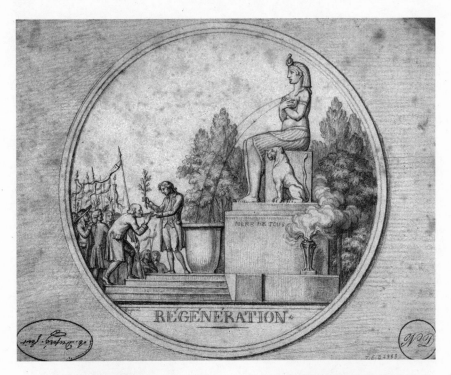

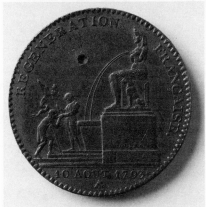

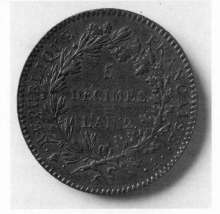

6.2a (top) *Fontaine de la Régénération*, Augustin Dupré, 1793.

6.2b (bottom, left) "Régénération française," five décime coin (front), Augustin Dupré, 1793.

6.2c (bottom, right) "Régénération française," five décime coin (back), Augustin Dupré, 1793.

between breastfeeding and feminism is far more complex than simple slogans or appeals to nature can capture. Until only the last one hundred or so years, when formula was invented, infant feeding required a mother (or at least a lactating person) to give her corporeal self in order to sustain the life of all humanity. According to Rousseau ([1762] 2011), not only life but a civilized political system depends on individual women feeding individual babies. Were mothers to abandon their babies in favour of a life of either hedonistic debauchery or unencumbered civic participation, there would be no human race. The women of the *querelle*, Rousseau, Wollstonecraft, Linneaus, and most intellectuals of the Enlightenment framed breastfeeding as a civic virtue, and yet Wollstonecraft's death fails to reject the hypothesis that maternal breastfeeding renders women no different from animals.

7 The Birth of the Breast versus Bottle Debates

If you are legal purists, you may wish me to change the title of this address to "Milk and Manslaughter," but if your lives were embittered as mine is, by seeing day after day this massacre of the innocents by unsuitable feeding, then I believe you would feel as I do that misguided propaganda on infant feeding should be punished as the most criminal form of sedition, and that these deaths should be regarded as murder.

Dr Cicely Williams, "Milk and Murder"

Infant formula is a modern invention that owes its existence to science and its promotion to the medical establishment. Nursing scholars Emily Stevens, Thelma Patrick, and Rita Pickler (2009) have traced its roots back to 1760, when Jean-Charles des Essartz examined the chemical composition of human milk and compared it to that produced by other members of the newly defined class *Mammalia*. In 1810, Nicholas Appert developed "a technique to sterilize food in sealed containers," and by 1835 evaporated milk in cans was patented; sugar was added in 1853 and the product sold as Eagle Brand Condensed Milk. The first powdered human milk substitute was patented in 1865 by Justus von Liebig, "consisting of cow's milk, wheat and malt flour, and potassium bicarbonate," beginning a trend that accelerated in the early twentieth century as scientists sought to develop a human milk substitute based first on cow's milk and then on soy or other milks for infants allergic to cow's milk. Although both the sweetened condensed milk and an unsweetened "evaporated milk" were highly popular for infant feeding and even recommended by pediatricians well into the 1930s and 1940s, none of these early "formulas" was safe for infants in terms of chemical composition, especially in contexts with poor sanitation (Stevens, Patrick, and Pickler 2009, 36).

Because these products were marketed as suitable alternatives but were not in fact safe for infant consumption, the early twentieth century saw the beginning of a public health movement to fight against the decline of breastfeeding, reminiscent of the eighteenth-century fight against wet nurses. According to historian and breastfeeding advocate Jacqueline Wolf,

> In the early 20th century, as part of the national campaign to lower infant mortality, public health officials around the country hung posters in urban neighborhoods urging mothers to breastfeed or to avoid feeding their babies the spoiled, adulterated cows' milk that pervaded US cities. The language on the posters was unambiguous. One commanded, "To lessen baby deaths let us have more mother-fed babies. You can't improve on God's plan. For your baby's sake – nurse it!" Another, which explained the importance of home pasteurization and keeping cows' milk on ice if a mother did not breastfeed, pleaded, "Give the Bottle-Fed Baby a Chance For Its Life!" (2003, 2000)

Despite the panicked tone of these entreaties, breastfeeding rates declined overall during this period, but so too did infant mortality rates. This was likely due, at least in part, to public health departments shifting their focus from promoting breastfeeding to promoting safe infant feeding practices more generally. According to Jacqueline Wolf, by the late 1920s, breastfeeding campaigns were replaced by "laws in most municipalities mandating the pasteurization and hygienic handling of cows' milk" (2003, 2000).

Further, new and improved formulations of breast milk alternatives quickly became readily available, riding a larger shift in cultural values that increasingly sought to create efficiencies in all areas of life through "modern" science (Nathoo and Ostry 2009). Physicians and scientists began to claim ownership over an area that had been the domain of women since the dawn of human evolution. Although men had long held opinions about infant feeding, in the 1920s male doctors named themselves the authorities on exactly how it should be done. Stevens, Patrick, and Pickler note,

> As formulas evolved and research supported their efficacy, manufacturers began to advertise directly to physicians. By 1929, the

American Medical Association (AMA) formed the Committee on Foods to approve the safety and quality of formula composition, forcing many infant food companies to seek AMA approval or the organization's "Seal of Acceptance." Three years later, advertising became regulated so that manufacturers could not solicit information to nonmedical personnel, which facilitated a positive relationship between physicians and formula companies. By the 1940s and 1950s, physicians and consumers regarded the use of formula as a well known, popular, and safe substitute for breastmilk. (2009, 36)

As breast milk alternatives became less likely to kill one's baby, fewer mothers engaged in the practice of breastfeeding. Simultaneously, women's participation in the paid labour force began to rise. During World War II, the need for women to enter the labour force became a matter of patriotic duty as men headed off to battle. At the war's end, women faced pressure to leave their jobs so that men could return to their pre-war jobs, especially those women who had entered into traditionally male-dominated manufacturing positions (Goldin and Olivetti 2013).

Although it is common today to speak of women "choosing" to stay home, from a sociological perspective it is important to consider the context within which individuals make their choices. From the early 1900s into the early 1950s, in the United States it was perfectly legal to discriminate against married women in hiring and even to fire women once they married (Goldin 1988). These employer policies, known as "marriage bars," created conditions that rendered it impossible for women to keep working in certain fields once they had married. These policies worked well for private firms and many school boards during the Depression years, when a steady supply of eager workers outnumbered the available jobs. Policies of rapid turnover served to suppress women's wages, in that women were unable to remain employed long enough to earn promotions or raises. At the same time, for Black women and other women of colour, "staying home" was an unavailable luxury. Given long-standing White supremacy, Black women and men alike were systematically kept out of more lucrative careers, with women typically relegated to domestic labour and physically demanding work in factories (Collins 2008).

Despite pressures on (at least White) women to stay home and raise families, women's overall labour-force participation rose steadily over the mid-twentieth century, and economists Stefania Albanesi and Claudia

Olivetti (2016) credit formula, along with innovations in reproductive medicine, with contributing to this shift. They point out that women's labour-force participation increased over the same years when birth rates were rising – the baby boom of 1930 to 1960. In other words, even though women were having more babies by mid-century, the availability of formula meant that they weren't the only ones who could feed them. Whether women's increasing participation in the workforce created a market for baby formula or the safety of formula allowed women to enter the labour force in greater numbers is a bit of a chicken-and-egg question. Either way, breastfeeding rates went into a free fall, with just 24.2 per cent of women even attempting to breastfeed and only 5.7 per cent of mothers breastfeeding for six months or longer by 1968.

It is difficult to obtain historical data on breastfeeding rates, but Lindsay Gartman Baker (2016), in her doctoral dissertation in economics, pieces together numerous data sets in order to plot breastfeeding rates in the twentieth-century United States. Included her analysis are responses to breastfeeding questions on a number of publicly available surveys, including the National Health Examination Survey (NHES), the National Fertility Survey (NFS), the National Health and Nutrition Examination Survey (NHANES), the National Survey of Family Growth (NSFG), and the National Health Interview Survey (NHIS). I plotted her data along with labour-force participation rates from the US Current Population Survey (US BLS 2020; US Bureau of the Census 1960) and infant mortality rates from the National Center for Health Statistics (CDC/NCHS 1967) and the UN Inter-agency Group for Child Mortality Estimation (UN IGME 2019).

As shown in figure 7.1, breastfeeding rates began to drop in 1940 and reached their nadir in the early 1970s, at which point they began to rise again. Interestingly, breastfeeding initiation rates were higher in 2016 (81.1 per cent) than they were in 1940 (72.1 per cent) despite a continued panic today that not enough mothers are breastfeeding. And this despite a revolutionary drop in the infant mortality rate from 47 per cent in 1940 to less than 6 per cent in 2016; the rate has been consistently under 10 per cent since 1989. While breastfeeding rates rapidly increased from the early 1970s, so did women's labour-force participation, plateauing and then declining starting in the early 2000s.

Formula manufacturers were all too ready to profit off of this shifting landscape (Freeman 2018). In the post-war era, manufacturers began marketing infant formula using scientific language suggesting that formula

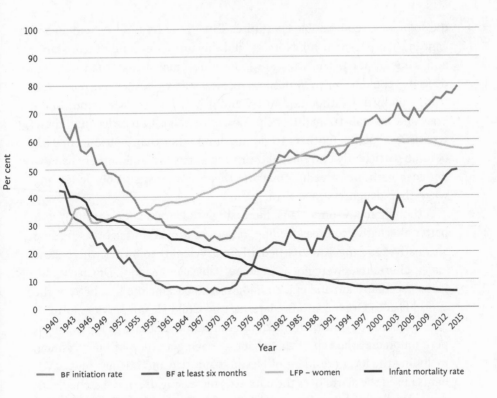

7.1 Breastfeeding initiation rates, rates of breastfeeding at least six months, women's labour-force participation rates, and infant mortality rates in the United States, 1940–2016.

was safer than breast milk, often including doctors' testimonials as to the products' safety. This mixing of medical advice with commercial interests was also seen in indirect ways, such as by surrounding magazine medical advice columns with formula milk advertisements (Nathoo and Ostry 2009). Although many corporations at the time focused their marketing on White audiences, canned milk companies targeted Black women in particular, as Black people migrated en masse from rural areas in the southern United States to factory jobs in cities in the northern United States. This migration meant that Black mothers had greater buying power and were likely unable to couple breastfeeding with their work (Freeman 2018).

Overall, increased medical management of women and infant health played out dramatically in obstetrics, beginning with the way that Western mothers gave birth. According to Nathoo and Ostry (2009), 35 per cent of Canadian mothers gave birth in a hospital in 1940 and nearly all mothers did so by 1960; comparable US statistics are 37 per cent in 1935 and 96 per cent in 1960 (Devitt 1977). Not only did this further expand doctor status and scope of practice (Carter 1995), but it also meant that infant feeding decisions could be made by hospital medical staff while mothers recovered from childbirth (Nathoo and Ostry 2009). With babies swept into nurseries and no staff trained to help mothers establish breastfeeding, there was little hope for mothers to do anything other than bottle-feed. This became particularly entrenched over time as fewer grandmothers had experience with breastfeeding, making them proponents of bottle-feeding when their daughters gave birth.

Although many physicians increasingly advocated for formula as a better alternative to breastfeeding, others continued to see breastfeeding alternatives as dangerous, particularly in developing countries where these "safer" alternatives were not as freely available. For instance, Dr Cicely Williams, a pediatrician and epidemiologist who became the first head of the World Health Organization's Maternal and Child Health Services in 1948, gave a talk in 1939 entitled "Milk and Murder" to a Rotary group in Singapore (quoted at the top of this chapter). Facing a group of businessmen, including the local president of Nestlé (Baumslag and Michels 1995), Williams raised the alarm over the country's increasing use of sweetened condensed milk over breastfeeding (Allain 1986). Today, this talk is still hailed by breastfeeding advocates for its uncompromising and pioneering condemnation of the decline in breastfeeding (UNICEF Innocenti Research Centre 2005). As featured on the arguably racist cover art of her reprinted speech (see figure 7.2), Williams stated that "Misguided propaganda on infant feeding should be punished as the most criminal form of sedition, and those deaths should be regarded as murder" (C. Williams [1939] 1986).

Williams, with her alarmist tone and her use of the word "sedition" ([1939] 1986, 5), suggests that not breastfeeding is not only dangerous for babies but also a threat to the authority of the state – as Rousseau argued two hundred years earlier. Her speech criticizes well-to-do mothers for being lazy and selfish, as did her eighteenth-century predecessor in philosophy, but her speech contains a notable difference from earlier thinkers. Rather than placing responsibility on individual women, Williams' ire was squarely aimed at social conditions and doctors' greed for hindering breastfeeding and causing infant death. Highlighting specific social inequalities in Singapore at that time, she made the point that wealthier bottle-fed infants were less likely to die than poor bottle-fed infants be-

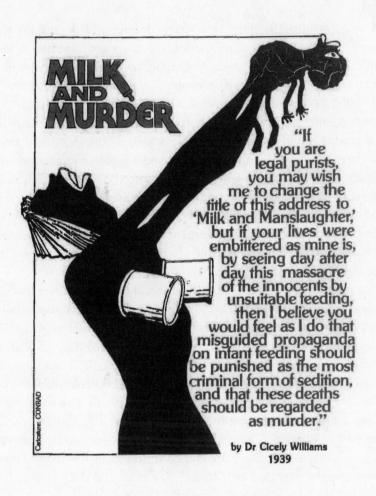

7.2 "Milk and Murder" reprint, 1986.

cause they had access to other advantages that made up for the ills caused by sweetened condensed milk. Thus, although her speech is often cited out of context, her solution to infant mortality from inadequate feeding supplements should not be oversimplified as "breast is best." Williams was in fact strongly advocating for improving the living conditions of poor mothers, which were so deplorable as to make it nearly impossible for them to breastfeed in the first place.

La Leche League and the Backlash against Working Women

In 1956, as breastfeeding rates were continuing a downward trend, a group of seven middle-class Catholic mothers got together in Franklin Park, Illinois, to found La Leche League, which remains the world's largest breastfeeding support organization today (Sandre-Pereira 2005). Though La Leche League is a secular organization with no official political stance on matters unrelated to breastfeeding, the religious background of the group's founders is unlikely a coincidence. Research has shown that "preference for Catholic religion" has had a negative impact on women's likelihood of participating in the labour force (Waite 1976, 78), and these mothers' Catholic beliefs are on display within La Leche League's maternalist and essentialist description of gender roles. For instance, until its most recent eighth edition, the organization's handbook, *The Womanly Art of Breastfeeding*, stressed the value of a male-breadwinner nuclear family as the ideal (Hausman 2003).

In emphasizing women's supposedly natural place as nurturers and child caregivers, the ideas of La Leche League initially resonated not only with Catholics but also with an emerging natural childbirth movement that had begun in the 1940s but took off in the 1970s. According to Nathoo and Ostry (2009), British obstetrician Dr Grantly Dick-Read (1944) unofficially started this movement with the publication of his book *Childbirth without Fear: The Principles and Practice of Natural Childbirth*. The book challenges hospital births as alienating and cold and became influential across Europe and North America. Coupled with La Leche League and the introduction of the "Lamaze technique" by French obstetrician Ferdinand Lamaze in the 1950s, the language of "natural" childbirth and child rearing contributed to a decade of highly circumscribed gender roles.

Among those urging women to focus on their gifts as caregivers to children were child development experts who argued that children needed their mothers to stay home with them (Waite 1976). Most famous among them was Dr Benjamin Spock, whose highly influential 1946 book *The Common Sense Book of Baby and Child Care* became the unofficial handbook of child-raising during the 1950s. According to nursing scholar and lactation consultant Diane Thulier (2009), Spock was an advocate for the advantages of breastfeeding in *principle*, although his advice, common for the period, often meant foreshortened breastfeeding in *practice*. For example, he encouraged a four-hour feeding schedule for babies in general and, "if a woman was suffering from 'even slightly sore' nipples" (Thulier 2009, 89), he recommended reducing nursing time to eight minutes per breast while supplementing with formula. As milk production is a result of demand and supply – the more you nurse, the more milk you produce – anyone involved in lactation support today will tell you that such advice is a recipe for insufficient milk and will likely lead to bottle-feeding.

Not only did Spock offer mixed support for breastfeeding, but he also framed such recommendations in an ideology of gender roles that saw women as best suited to domestic life and men to paid labour. Among his advice was the following:

> It would save money in the end if the government paid a com-
> fortable allowance to all mothers (of young children) who would
> otherwise be compelled to work. You can think of it this way: useful,
> well-adjusted citizens are the most valuable possession a country
> has, and good mother care during early childhood is the surest way
> to produce them. It doesn't make sense to let mothers go to work
> making dresses in factories or tapping typewriters in offices, and
> have them pay other people to do a poorer job of bringing up their
> children. (Spock 1946, 484, quoted in Waite 1976, 77)

As Waite notes, in research discussed in the previous section, the steepest drop in labour-force participation took place among women most likely to read books on expert advice: the highly educated.

Waite's (1976) findings are similar to research I carried out with Mary C. Noonan examining the impact of breastfeeding on women's earnings (Rippeyoung and Noonan 2012b). We used the US National Longitudinal Survey of Youth data, a representative sample of US men and women aged fourteen to twenty-two years in 1979, to compare the income trajectories between mothers who breastfed for six months or longer (the recommended duration), for less than six months, or not at all. Using linear growth models, we were able to compare not just the incomes of the different mothers but each mother's ups and downs in earnings over time, from the year before they gave birth until five years after. As shown in figure 7.3, what we found was that though both short-duration and long-duration breastfeeders start with similar incomes, over time the mothers doing the recommended six months of breastfeeding experience steeper declines in earnings. Although the main reason for this is that they were more likely

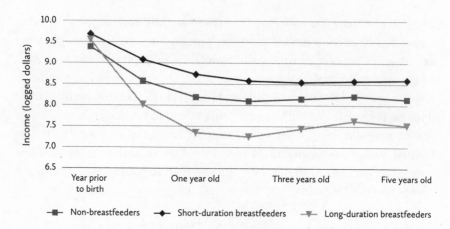

7.3 Logged income trajectories of long-duration breastfeeders (six months or longer), short-duration breastfeeders (less than six months), and non-breastfeeders (labelled incorrectly in the original source as "formula feeders").

to reduce their work hours or exit the labour force entirely, we controlled for their work commitment prior to motherhood, which means that the results do not reflect differing levels of commitment to working by breast-feeding status. In other words, breastfeeding poses a real dilemma for those who want to do "right" by breastfeeding as they are likely to be financially penalized when they do so, and this is especially true for professional and highly educated women.

Women's Bodies and Women's Liberation

Highly educated women were also those most influenced by the 1963 publication of Betty Friedan's *The Feminine Mystique* (Nathoo and Ostry 2009). Focusing nearly exclusively on the concerns of well-educated, primarily White middle- and upper-class women, Friedan ([1963] 2010) challenged the 1950s promise of domestic bliss for women. As she wrote,

> Over and over again, stories in women's magazines insist that
> women can know fulfillment only at the moment of giving birth to
> a child. They deny the years when she can no longer look forward
> to giving birth, even if she repeats the act over and over again. In
> the feminine mystique, there is no other way for a woman to dream
> of creation or of the future. There is no other way she can even

dream about herself, except as her children's mother, her husband's wife. (115)

Friedan went on to help form and to serve as first president of the National Organization for Women (NOW) in 1966. Daphne Spain describes the organization:

Open both to men and women and patterned after the National Association for the Advancement of Colored People [NAACP], its membership was predominantly middle aged, middle class, and white. At its first national convention in 1967 NOW issued a Bill of Rights with eight demands: passage of the Equal Rights Amendment [ERA]; enforcement of the law banning sex discrimination in employment; maternity leave rights in employment and in social security benefits; tax deductions for home and child-care expenses for working parents; child day-care centers (established by law on the same basis as parks, libraries, and public schools); equal and unsegregated education; equal job training opportunities and allowance for women in poverty; and the right of women to control their reproductive lives. (2011, 156)

Although Friedan has since been criticized for essentializing the experiences of a particular class of mothers as representative of all mothers, her work nonetheless laid bare the experience of women who had grown disillusioned with the promises of domesticity that had failed to materialize for them in the 1950s. The idealization of women's "natural" role in society was as frustrating to housewives of the 1950s as it had been to the women of the *querelle des femmes*, providing a flashpoint for the women's movement of the 1960s as larger and more diverse groups of women challenged the notion that women's greatest satisfaction could be found in service to their husbands, children, and families.

Although Friedan sparked a more privileged group of women to leave their homes and start agitating, the larger movement for women's liberation emerged in a context of pre-existing Black civil rights and Black women's social justice, along with labour and anti-war movements. Although White, middle-class women dominated NOW, many early organizers were Black women frustrated with the hostility to feminism they experienced in the civil rights movement. However, their frustration eventually turned to NOW for focusing almost exclusively on the ERA and ignoring issues that Black members felt were more pressing in their communities. As such, the organization's second president, Aileen Hernandez, left NOW to form the National Black Feminist Organization (NBFO) in 1973, along with Eleanor Holmes Norton, Alice Walker, Shirley Chisholm, and Barbara Smith, among others (Spain 2011). A smaller group within the NBFO, led by Barbara Smith, then split off to found the Combahee River Collective in Boston (named for the site of the Civil War battle planned and led by Harriet Tubman on 2 June 1863). According to Spain, their self-titled manifesto, published in 1976, "came to define black feminism" (2011, 157). Within the pages of the manifesto, the Combahee River Collective took aim at the explicit sexism within Black liberation movements, the racism in mainstream women's organizing like NOW, and the heterosexism embedded within the capitalist system that undergirded the oppression of all peoples. They advocated for a politics that focuses on one's own oppression under the notion of the personal being political. They sought a politics of transformation through "a healthy love for ourselves, our sisters and our community." In addition, they wrote that they "believe that the most profound and potentially most radical politics come directly out of our own identity, as opposed to working to end somebody else's oppression" (Combahee River Collective 1976, 4). Importantly, this politics, based on the humble assertion of equal value, was not rooted in individualism. Rather, the collective argued,

> We realize that the liberation of all oppressed peoples necessitates the destruction of the political-economic systems of capitalism and imperialism as well as patriarchy. We are socialists because we believe that work must be organized for the collective benefit of those who do the work and create the products, and not for the profit of the bosses. Material resources must be equally distributed among those who create these resources. We are not convinced, however, that a socialist revolution that is not also a feminist and anti-racist revolution will guarantee our liberation. (5)

During this heady time of political activism and intersecting social movements, a new women's health movement also emerged, as best exemplified in the creation of the Boston Women's Health Collective and the publication of the booklet *Women and Their Bodies* in 1970. This health manifesto would later be expanded into the influential and comprehen-sive guide to women's health *Our Bodies, Ourselves* (BWHBC and Norsigian 2011) still in print today. The collective's origins are outlined on its website:

> In May of 1969, as the women's movement was gaining momentum and influence in the Boston area and elsewhere around the world, 12 women ranging in age from 23 to 39 met during a women's liberation conference at Emmanuel College. In a workshop on "Women and their Bodies," they shared information and discussed their experien-ces with doctors.
>
> The discussions were so provocative and fulfilling that they formed the Doctor's Group, the forerunner to the Boston Women's Health Book Collective, which later changed to Our Bodies Our-selves, to find out more about their bodies, their lives, their sexual-ity and relationships, and to talk with each other about what they learned. ("Our Story" n.d.)

This radical organization's first typewritten and stapled publication was presented as a "course" to empower women to have greater control over their bodies through greater knowledge. The collective advocated sex for pleasure and access to abortion as part of women's comprehensive health-care rights, framing women's struggles with their health as connected to larger capitalist and patriarchal ideologies of control. As they write,

> Marcuse says that "health is a state defined by an elite." A year ago few of us understood this statement. What does he mean? We believed that all people want to be healthy and that some of us are more fortunate than others because we have more competent doctors. "Now you should go to Dr. A. Man. He's my doctor and he's just great!"
>
> Today we understand the stark truth of Marcuse's statement. We have not only started to look at health differently, but we have found that health is one more example of the many problems we as people, especially as women, face in this society. We have not had power to determine medical priorities; they are determined by the corporate medical industry (including drug companies, Blue Cross, the AMA and other profit-making groups) and academic research. We have learned that we are not to blame for choosing a bad doctor or not

having the money to choose. Certainly, some doctors have learned medical skills better than others, but how good are technical skills if they are not practiced in a human way?

We as women are redefining competence: a doctor who behaves in a male chauvinist way is not competent, even if he has medical skills. We have decided that health can no longer be defined by an elite group of white, upper middle-class men. It must be defined by us, the women who need the most health care, in a way that meets the needs of all our sisters and brothers – poor, black, brown, red, yellow and pink. (BWHC 1970, 6)

They go on to explore the ways in which the medical profession has been used to control women and keep them in a position of submission, both in its treatment of women and through what classical sociology theorist Max Weber might call "social closure." Social closure is the process whereby professionals limit entry into the profession through higher education and testing and by using mystifying language in order to make their knowledge inaccessible to the general public and in turn make it easier for them to demand a higher reward for their expertise. The booklet *Women and Their Bodies* continues,

Perhaps the most obvious indication of this ideology is the way that doctors treat us as women patients. We are considered stupid, mind-less creatures, unable to follow instructions (known as orders). While men patients may also be treated this way, we fare worse because women are thought to be incapable of understanding or dealing with our own situation. Health is not something which belongs to a person, but is rather a precious item that the doctor doles out from his stores. Thus, the doctor preserves his expertise and powers for himself. (BWHC 1970, 6)

The collective's radical feminist agenda did not end with challenges to the healthcare system alone, either. They argued that "knowledge of our reproductive organs is vital to overcome objectification" (BWHC 1970, 10) as part of a larger liberation program that could liberate all people. They saw that the greatest threats to human health were not the doctors or the healthcare system itself but rather a capitalist system that is outside the control of any individuals. They pointed to lead paint in slum housing, hookworm in the rural South, coal mines, industrial working conditions, the failure to provide preventive medical care, and doctors' refusal to participate in a free vaccination program as contributing to the state of health care in the United States. As an alternative, they lauded the Soviet Union's healthcare system for offering medical care regardless of ability to pay and the Black Panther Party of Boston for setting "up a free clinic in Roxbury on the pattern of the Judson Mobile Health unit in NY in which patients are encouraged to ask questions, and are invited to look through microscopes at their own blood samples, and participate in the decision making" (189). They went on to caution readers to be careful about harassment, however, as "the Free Clinic in Berkeley was attacked by the Berkeley Police with canisters of CS gas during a fight over People's Park. One of the Canisters was shot through the window of the clinic during regular clinic hours. CS is a dangerous substance, especially when used against already sick people" (189–90).

Clearly, efforts to inform and disseminate knowledge about health were seen as a threat to authority. This isn't surprising, considering that these health movements themselves saw increasing understanding about one's body as part of a larger educational and justice-fighting agenda to dismantle capitalist and patriarchal control of the bodies of workers, women, and Black people and other people of colour.

As mentioned in chapter 2, it is interesting to note that breastfeeding was not a subject of significant interest in *Women and Their Bodies*. In fact, the booklet mentions the practice just twice. First, it refers to "care of the nipples: little attention is required beyond simple cleanliness. If the nipples become sore a nipple shield may be used temporarily. If your doctor is not helpful with nursing problems call La Leche League" (BWHC 1970, 174). A few pages later it states, "If you're planning to breastfeed your baby – read some good, supportive books about it first. *Commonsense Childbirth* has an excellent section on breastfeeding, as does the Kitzinger book, and Karen Pryor's. Don't let people discourage you, and remember that sleep and lots of liquids are necessary" (177).

Interesting to our purposes here, breastfeeding was not put forth as a feminist cause to rally around by any of these feminist groups or leaders. Unlike the women of the *querelle*, or Mary Wollstonecraft, these feminists were decidedly opposed to the use of women's bodies to signal women's greater virtues. However, it is interesting to me that this also suggests a kind of uncertainty about how to theorize breastfeeding as a feminist cause, much to the frustration of many feminist breastfeeding advocates, as discussed in chapter 2.

Is Infant Formula Actually Risky for Babies?

Unlike the laissez-faire attitude of *Women and Their Bodies*, current discussions about breastfeeding now tend to be presented as a crisis that needs solving. As will be discussed later, even among the feminist breastfeeding promoters, the foundation for breastfeeding as a feminist cause is the belief in the superior benefits of breast milk for mothers and babies (Smith 2018). This is likely why there was such a brouhaha when Joan Wolf (2013) suggested that the scientific evidence on the benefits of breast milk is weak. However, in my own experience as a researcher, I discovered an incredibly obvious but never discussed problem in the science suggesting that formula is risky for infants – the hinted-at finding that led a lactivist to email me (see chapter 2): although heaps of research exist showing health differences between breastfed and not-breastfed babies, what "not breastfed" means is rarely explored or differentiated.

My and my co-authors' review of the literature identifies a consistent lack of attention to precisely what babies are being fed as alternatives to breast milk (Rippey, Aravena, and Nyonator 2020). Instead, researchers appear to assume that when babies are not breastfed, they are fed only formula – despite the very real possibility that non-breastfed infants are being fed other supplemental foods, like cow's or other animal milk, cereals, soups, or other foods, that are known to be harmful (Norris et al. 2003; Tarini et al. 2006). Even Mary Noonan and I made this mistake in our paper that I discussed above (Rippeyoung and Noonan 2012b), including the published key for our graph, by incorrectly identifying the non-breastfed infants as "formula fed." In the data we were using, women were simply asked if babies were breastfed, and we just assumed that those who said they didn't breastfeed were formula-feeding their babies. However, babies are fed lots of foods that are neither human breast milk nor formula, all of which are bad for the infant gut.

I didn't even realize this was a mistake until a few years after our paper was published when I started working on a separate project about breastfeeding in Indonesia. Because I didn't read Indonesian, and there is not a lot published on the feminist politics of breastfeeding in Indonesia (at least at that time), I widened my literature review to include more studies of basic health and science than I normally would focus on. In the process of reviewing these articles, most of which were unrelated to my question, I stumbled across one that blew my mind (although I cannot, for the life of me, find it! It is like a mythical paper that came to give me a message and then disappeared). In the paper, as I recall, the authors were interested in understanding how well mothers were practising exclusive breastfeeding. What they found was that all the mothers said that they were exclusively breastfeeding, but when they were asked a follow-up question – "So, when did you start giving your baby banana?" – many mothers said something to the effect of "oh, when he was first born, he was very hungry." Later, when I finally travelled to Indonesia, I discovered that this is actually quite a common practice: to feed babies, sometimes on the day of their birth, bananas mashed with the liquid from cooking rice. Similarly, one of the mothers I interviewed in my lesbian study was a third-generation Mexican American who spoke of the frustration she felt from her family who tried (unsuccessfully) to convince her to feed her newborn a soup traditional in their community consisting of ground beef, flour, and water. We sort of chuckled at the time in our interview over the phone at how gross and strange that sounded, but in hindsight, this kind of thing started to sound both common and really scary.

As I started to pore over scientific research and popular recommendations about the risks of formula and sought out any data I could find to see how "not breastfed" was measured, I realized that no one was paying much attention to this. A lot of attention has been given to making sure that "exclusive breastfeeding" is measured carefully. According to international lactation consultant Helen Armstrong, in a guest editorial in the *Journal of Human Lactation* back in 1991 about consistency in breastfeeding definitions, "lactation consultants regularly encounter published studies in which the category *breastfed* indiscriminately groups together children receiving relatively few breastfeeds (and assorted supplements or interferences) and exclusively or substantially breastfed. Haphazardness in the definition of breastfeeding has made much in the existing literature inconclusive" (1991, 51). Around the same time, the Interagency Group for Action on Breastfeeding created a standardized schema for defining breastfeeding in order to provide consistent measurements and improve comparability between studies (Labbok and Krasovec 1990). This schema, categorizing breastfeeding on a scale from no breastfeeding to exclusive breastfeeding with no supplements, was adopted by the WHO in

1990 and is used in most breastfeeding health studies today (Lamberti et al. 2011).

Although there is nothing in this schema that suggests whether or how to measure what those "supplements" are, pressure has been increasing to shift infant feeding rhetoric from the notion that "breast is best" to the idea that formula is dangerous. For instance, in its "14 Risks of Formula Feeding" brochure, the Infant Feeding Action Coalition (INFACT) Canada (n.d.) lists the following risks: lung infections, ear infections, chronic diseases, effects of environmental poisons, allergy, asthma, heart disease, death from diseases, obesity, childhood cancers, diarrhea, diabetes, infection from contaminated formula, and lower intelligence in infants. Breastfeeding advocate James Akre (2010) has suggested that the dangers of formula are so great that a "counterrevolution" against the tide of formula needs to be won. Suggestions for winning this counterrevolution have included making formula available only with a doctor's prescription or in emergency situations, or by instituting a luxury tax on formula (Akre 2010; Baumslag and Michels 1995).

Others have critiqued public health efforts that discuss the benefits of breastfeeding on the grounds that they implicitly normalize formula. For example, Alison Stuebe argues, "public health campaigns and medical literature have traditionally described the 'benefits of breastfeeding,' comparing health outcomes among breastfed infants against a reference group of formula-fed infants. Although mathematically synonymous with reporting the 'risk of not breastfeeding,' this approach implicitly defines formula feeding as the norm" (2009, 223). Stuebe's claim that formula feeding is "mathematically synonymous" with not breastfeeding would only be true if "not breastfed" infants were fed *only* formula. However, in the studies she cites (Cushing et al. 1998; Duncan et al. 1993; Pisacane et al. 2010; Quigley, Kelly, and Sacker 2007), the reference group is "not breastfed," not "formula fed." Similarly, Melinda McNiel, Miriam Labbok, and Sheryl Abrahams (2010) examined research studies on eight childhood conditions and assessed how breastfeeding was measured and health outcomes. They were careful only to evaluate "studies that reported 'exclusively breastfed,' 'fully breastfed,' or 'totally breastfed' as a comparison group. *Lack of exclusive breastfeeding in developed countries is an appropriate proxy indicator of formula feeding* [my italics]" (51). In other words, they assumed that any children not fed breast milk were formula fed.

Despite the significant advances in the quality of breast milk alternatives since the early days of sweetened condensed milk, research into formula's relative safety has been, for the most part, completely missing. Around 2014, Fabiola Aravena, John Paul Nyonator, and I began to carry out research to compare the health impacts of breast milk versus formula, rather than breast milk versus anything else. Given that research clearly shows that feeding complementary or supplemental foods before four to six months of age makes babies sick, we wondered if there was widespread omitted-variable bias in breastfeeding research. In other words, we wanted to know if properly prepared formula itself is dangerous or if some of the "non-breastfed" babies were actually being fed things like Hamburger Helper soup.

The results of our analysis showed that once one we controlled for the premature introduction of complementary foods (anything other than formula before four months of age), there were no significant differences between purely formula-fed and exclusively breastfed infants' likelihood of being hospitalized, prescribed antibiotics or other medicine, or contracting a fever or diarrhea. Babies fed formula, even if partially breastfed, however, do have higher rates of hard stool and cough/wheeze. Going against everything in the literature (and tested and retested in various permutations over the years we worked on this), mixed-fed babies (those fed both formula and breast milk) actually had lower rates of diarrhea and runny nose or cold than exclusively breastfed babies. Now, before any formula feeders get too excited, remember that this is one study on one data set and that exclusively breastfed babies are clearly less likely to get hard stool or cough or wheeze. And, in the context of COVID-19, we know that cough and wheeze or other respiratory ailments can be deadly. Further, the data were based on parental reports, and one mom's definition of diarrhea (a potentially fatal ailment in infants) could be another mom's "watery stool" (a common description of normal breastfed babies' poo).

But still, one would think that the mere observation that no one is attending to the measurement of "not breastfed" would be considered an important omission to be rectified. At the very least, this might pique the curiosity of researchers, assuming they are interested in pursuing the scientific goal of falsifying claims and not simply on an ideological crusade to get kids breastfeeding no matter the science. However, our experience in seeking publication of our article raised some serious doubts about that assumption. My co-authors were students of mine – one in sociology, the other in population health – and I had published in multiple reputable journals by the time we began submitting the paper. I had also been teaching quantitative methods for nearly a decade, had supervised undergraduate and graduate theses using various statistical analyses, and had graduated from arguably one of the top graduate departments in social statistics in the United States, the University of Iowa. Iowa, though best known for its creative writing program, was remarkable in its sociology department for being nearly exclusively populated with quantitative researchers, themselves trained at the very top quantitative programs in the country. In our analysis, my co-authors and I paid careful attention to measurement, using advanced statistical methods (first logistic regression, then logistic with generalized estimating equations) on a large, longitudinal data set collected by the US Food and Drug Administration (FDA) and the Centers for Disease Control and Prevention (CDC). Despite our credentials and the important implications of our research, our study was rejected by ten different academic journals before finding a home at the *Journal of Pediatric Gastroenterology and Nutrition* (Rippey, Aravena, and Nyonator 2020).

As sociologists, we first submitted the paper to three sociology of health journals; none wanted to publish it, and all suggested it was more appropriate for a public health journal. After a few failed tries in public health we changed course and began submitting to medical journals. We did get one editor who let us rewrite it to make it sound "less biased" before she would consider sending it to reviewers but then rejected it. Some versions of our paper may have been rejected owing to stylistic differences between health and social science journals, which took us a bit of time to get the hang of, and earlier versions of the paper involved less sophisticated statistical methods. I had naïvely thought that the paper would be seen as groundbreaking, as it is exceedingly rare to identify an omitted variable in decades of research on a subject that no one else noticed.

In one bout of frustration, I obliquely shared about the research on Twitter, leading a few interested people to ask me for more info. But I was afraid of getting scooped because I wanted us to be the first ones to publish this idea, assuming the paper would be huge. My other reason for not wanting to share our results was that I did not want to advertise the results before the paper went through peer review; to be sure we weren't missing some key variable ourselves. A few people reached out, wanting to read it, and I thankfully relented to two health experts in exchange for any feedback they might have to offer. One, a scholar in pediatric public health, and the other, a pediatric nutritionist with an MD, both reviewed the paper and responded first with something along the lines of "wow!" The MD noted that she had no idea that so many parents were feeding their kids something other than formula and so she was going to start asking her patients about this explicitly in her practice.

They also offered some extremely helpful suggestions for reframing the paper for revision. In particular, one suggested changing it from comparing formula feeding to breastfeeding infants to comparing infants fed complementary foods to those fed nothing but breast milk or formula. The difference statistically was negligible, but rhetorically it was huge. I was a bit disappointed in my heart because we all know that complementary foods are unhealthy for babies and I feared there would not be a sizable enough contribution to the literature within this framework. However, somewhat miraculously, I discovered that the European Society for Paediatric Gastroenterology, Hepatology and Nutrition (ESPGHAN) Committee on Nutrition had published a paper saying that research had not assessed whether complementary foods had different effects on breastfed versus formula-fed infants (Fewtrell et al. 2017). With this new hook to frame our paper, we submitted to the flagship journal of the ESPGHAN (and the North American SPGHAN), the *Journal of Pediatric Gastroenterology and Nutrition*, and it was accepted with minimal revisions. The journal even invited us to create supplemental materials for doctors to get continuing medical education (CME) credits for reading the paper. We were thrilled. I tweeted about it and awaited the controversy. A few people in my Twitter circles liked it and were excited to read it, but not much happened. Since I'd tweeted it around Christmas, I figured I would tweet about it again in a long thread a few weeks later. Meh ... radio silence. Nobody seemed to care much. Huh.

What's particularly disturbing to me is that a 2018 status report from the WHO showed that 99 per cent of global policies that limit the marketing of breast milk substitutes target infant formula, whereas only 44 per cent target complementary foods. If premature introduction of complementary foods is unquestionably harmful to infants, why are we not putting more effort into stopping that? If our concern is truly about infant health, shouldn't we even consider providing free or subsidized formula to mothers who are unable to breastfeed, to ensure that babies are not being fed thinned porridges because of the exorbitant cost of formula?

Is There Really No Difference between Formula and Breast Milk?

I want to be clear that even if research to date has fallen prey to omitted-variable bias, formula and breast milk are not the same. In their review of the literature, Christine Dieterich et al. (2013) suggest that human milk confers health benefits to infants from its antibody secretory IgA (sIgA) and from monoglycerides and medium- and long-chain fatty acids with antimicrobial properties that protect the gastrointestinal tract from the adherence of pathogens. Human milk is also found to synthesize "several essential micronutrients, namely vitamins B12, B6, folate, and vitamin K" (35), which not only help with infant growth but also protect babies' vulnerable immune systems. Lactoferrin in breast milk is said to increase the functional ability of infant bodies to digest iron. Further, "hormones, neuropeptides, and growth factors" (35) found in breast milk, such as leptin and ghrelin, may help in the self-regulation of food intake in breastfed babies. And, importantly, all the mounds and mounds of research showing that breastfed babies do better than infants fed "just whatever" is not wrong. Early supplemental foods clearly make babies sick, and from a public health perspective, if you want to ensure the healthiest outcomes for the most children around the world, exclusive breastfeeding is a very safe bet. However, our one study (Rippey, Aravena, and Nyonator 2020) seems to suggest that properly prepared formula without any supplemental foods for the first six months is a pretty safe bet too. What is more important about the study than our particular findings are the questions it raises.

The results suggest that the reason non-breastfed infants have worse outcomes than their breastfed peers might have a lot to do with the high cost of infant formula and the many pressures and forces confronting lower-income women. The people most likely to give non-formula and non-breast milk to babies are poor mothers who struggle to pay for formula, the cost of which can add up to over a thousand dollars a year. Much research has shown that breastfed infants tend to be in families with higher levels of education and earnings (Heck et al. 2006), despite the fact that formula is a far more expensive substance than human milk, not including the costs of women's time (Rippeyoung and Noonan 2012b). In their study of recipients of the Special Supplemental Nutrition Program for Women, Infants, and Children (WIC), Fornasaro-Donahue et al. (2014) found that all formula-feeding mothers indicated buying additional formula on top of what was supplied by WIC but that 10 per cent of mothers nonetheless reported purchasing an amount of formula inadequate to meet their infants' needs. Drawing on past research, the authors note that

> Previous research shows that early introduction of complementary foods (weaning) is associated with young maternal age, low maternal education, low socioeconomic status, absence or short duration of breastfeeding, maternal smoking, and lack of information or advice from health care providers. Early introduction of cow's milk is associated with low maternal education and low socioeconomic status. About one third of American infants are exposed to unmodified milk before 12 months of age, and one third [of all infants] are introduced to complementary foods before 4 months. Because the mothers in this study were of low socioeconomic background, it is possible that some of these mothers were supplementing their infants with complementary foods and/or unmodified cow's milk. These practices may contribute to the adverse health consequences associated with formula feeding in low-income populations. (567)

This speculation is consistent with Frank's (2020) findings in research exploring infant food security in Canada. She found that access to affordable formula for non-breastfed infants was often extremely difficult for the low-income mothers she interviewed. With limited funds, some mothers turned to supplementary foods for their hungry babies when their formula ran out.

However, regardless of class, Fein and Falci (1999) found that in the United States, rates of the premature introduction of supplemental foods were high across economic classes. Based on self-reports by mothers in the FDA's Infant Feeding Practices Study, at two months of age, 35 per cent of formula-fed babies had other food added to their bottles, and 21 per cent had cereal added to their bottles. Adjusted percentages showed that younger mothers (ages twelve to twenty-four) were twice as likely as mothers thirty-five years and older to add cereal to their formula-fed babies' bottles (21 per cent versus 9 per cent) (Fein and Falci 1999). Similarly, using the 2002 Feeding Infants and Toddlers Study (FITS), Briefel et al. found that "about 29% of all infants were introduced to infant cereals or pureed foods before four months of age" (2004, S33).

Considering that formula can be expensive and that foods can be added only to a bottle (not to a breast), logically one would expect that formula-fed infants would be more likely to be prematurely introduced to supplemental foods than breastfed infants. Further, considering the health costs of early supplemental food introduction, logically one would expect to see more illness in formula-fed infants. However, the illness would be due to the supplemental foods, rather than the formula itself. Hence, this is why we carried out our analysis and in fact found this to be the case.

Formula isn't necessarily risky, but complementary foods certainly are. And babies fed formula are far more likely to be given complementary foods. In our analyses, in fact, we found that at two months, fewer than 2 per cent of breastfed infants were given complementary foods such as baby cereal or pureed fruits and vegetables, while around half of formula-fed infants were given such foods (Rippey, Aravena, and Nyonator 2020). All of which raises the question: Shouldn't global health efforts aimed at improving outcomes for infants be more concerned about improving the safety of infant formula feeding? Or, perhaps this underscores the connection between breastfeeding promotion and deeper convictions about women's moral or natural responsibility to limit their aspirations to the care and feeding of their families.

8 Breastfeeding as a Solution to Global Problems

A whole generation of Third World mothers is virtually giving up breast-feeding and turning to powdered milk formula because of the crass marketing practices of profit-hungry companies like Nestlé. A whole generation of their children will, if they live, grow up physically weak and mentally retarded.

It may be too late for them, but it's not too late for babies yet unborn.

You can help. Please help. Please, please join today and send a check for as much as you possibly can spare ... and then some.

Douglas A. Johnson, national chairperson,
Infant Feeding Action Coalition

As discussed in the previous chapter, and bluntly summarized by international breastfeeding experts and advocates Naomi Baumslag and Dia Michels, until the twentieth century, babies who weren't breastfed "died like flies" (1995, 113) and thus there has been money to be made in the development of breast milk substitutes. In response to the commercialization of infant feeding, getting more women to breastfeed has been a central part of global hunger efforts since the 1970s. This was perhaps most dramatically implemented in 2009 when Indonesia enacted a law mandating exclusive breastfeeding for six months, only to be outdone in 2014 when the United Arab Emirates (UAE) mandated two *years* of breastfeeding. Sultan al-Sammahi of the UAE federal national council was quoted in the *Guardian* as saying, "This is the right of every child for two years ... [I]f they do not have a mother or have been neglected, then they should get this right from someone else" (Graham-Harrison 2014). In other words, infants have a right to obtain a wet nurse. The article quotes another council member, Ahmad al-Shamsi, who "said the law aimed to make breastfeeding 'a duty and not an option' for able mothers. 'This is part of raising a child. This is mandatory,' he said. 'Laws are not all about fines and penalties – some are also humane'" (Graham-Harrison 2014). Although the UAE law has received little attention from the field of breastfeeding promotion, the Indonesian law has been viewed either uncritically or positively as evidence of support for women and a strike against nefarious formula makers (WHO 2014).

I argue, however, that many of the actors behind these movements were neither feminist nor progressive, and much of the global concern with infant feeding has been driven by organizations and people in support of the broader political and economic trend known as neoliberalism. As defined by Nik-Khah and Van Horn (2016), neoliberalism welcomes "free market" capitalism and favours individual-level solutions rather than addressing the roots of inequality at the societal or global levels. In this way, global breastfeeding campaigns have provided countries and corporations with a means to absolve themselves of responsibility for the exploitation of local resources and people by locating the solution to the problems they created within the power of women's breasts.

The Evolution of Global Breastfeeding Policy

In 1974, the worldwide decline in breastfeeding rates was a major focus of the 27th World Health Assembly of the United Nations World Health Organization. Three years later, a worldwide boycott of Nestlé erupted in protest of the unethical marketing practices of formula manufacturers in developing countries. This led the WHO to introduce the International Code of Marketing of Breast-milk Substitutes in 1981, which advocated strict guidelines for formula labelling, prohibited providing free samples of formula in healthcare settings, and banned sales incentives for formula marketers. Every country assembled at the 37th World Health Assembly in Switzerland signed on to the code, with one exception: the United States, which continues to reject the code today (Jacobs 2018).

As with any international agreement, the WHO Code had no enforcement mechanism behind it, only the power of its authors' rhetoric. Thus, upon its ratification, WHO director-general Dr Halfdan Mahler of Denmark appealed to the delegates to enact local legislation in support of the code. Interestingly, he drew on Jean-Jacques Rousseau's notion of the social contract. Speaking before the assembled delegates, Mahler stated,

More than 200 years ago Jean-Jacques Rousseau, citizen of this very Geneva in which this Health Assembly takes place, described the nature of such a social contract. Now listen to how he described it: "A form of association which defends and protects with the whole force of the community the person and property of every associate and by means of which each coalescing with all, nevertheless obeys only himself and remains as free as before." (WHA 1981, 17)

He went on to argue, "Health is a fundamental human right" (17), but this right comes with responsibilities for individuals and for states. Urging action, Mahler stated that all of the code's signers "are expected to adopt the strategy at the highest political level and to ensure the means for implementing it. But at the same time they are expected to give people the right to assume growing responsibility for their own health and they are expected to help them to generate the means to do so" (18). He went on to quote Rousseau again: "The citizens being all equal by the social contract, what all ought to do all can prescribe, while no one has the right to demand that another should do what he will not do himself" (18). Mahler's use of "all" and "himself" is interesting, given that the subject at hand is an activity performed nearly exclusively by women. His words, in addition to the vast efforts of those in support of the code, have been extremely influential. According to a report produced by the WHO, UNICEF, and the International Baby Food Action Network (IBFAN), "As of 2018 a total of 35 countries have full Code provisions covered in law, while 31 have legal measures with many Code provisions in place, and 70 have legal measures incorporating few code provisions in law" (WHO 2018, 11). The most comprehensive legislation can be found in South-East Asian and African countries, while Europe and the Americas have enacted the fewest measures (WHO 2018).

Commerciogenic Malnutrition and the Nestlé Boycott

This sea change towards breastfeeding-focused global health policy sought to address the more egregious tactics with which infant formula is marketed in low-income countries (a.k.a. the "developing world"). Given inadequate access to electricity, refrigeration, and clean water, breastfeeding would seem logically safer than expensive products that require caution in preparation, handling, and storage. A further problem with marketing tactics such as giving out free samples has to do with the fact that breastfeeding works through supply and demand: the more a mother nurses, the more milk she produces. Thus, if a mother feeds her baby from cans of free formula for too many days in a row, she may lose her milk supply entirely. Even supplementing one's breast milk with formula can reduce milk production, putting infants at risk if their families cannot afford to continue to purchase these expensive products (Baumslag and Michels 1995).

In response to these concerns, global health scholar and pediatrician Dr Derrick Jelliffe introduced the term "commerciogenic malnutrition" in the 1970s to highlight the plight of infants who were fed insufficient and unsafe alternatives to breast milk (Jelliffe 1972; Jelliffe and Jelliffe 1977). This inspired the British charity War on Want to publish a report called "The Baby Killer" in the *New Internationalist* (Muller 1974). This report, along with the 1975 documentary film *Bottle Babies* (Krieg 1975), raised international awareness about the problem of predatory marketing of infant milk substitutes. When "The Baby Killer" was translated into German with the new title "Nestlé Kills Babies," worldwide boycotts and protests singled out Nestlé, which responded with a libel suit against the German publisher of the translated version (Baumslag and Michels 1995).

Although the *New Internationalist* is on the left of the political spectrum, the Nestlé boycott transcended political boundaries. In fact, according to Rita Catherine Murphy (2012), in her master's thesis about the anti-Nestlé Infant Feeding Action Coalition (INFACT), influential figures in the Catholic Church were among those interested in addressing infant feeding as an international crisis. For example, the Sisters of the Precious Blood launched a lawsuit against Bristol-Myers for marketing infant formula in developing countries. Murphy also identifies other Catholic Church connections:

> It was my mother, Donna Murphy, who first informed me of the existence of the Nestlé boycott. Throughout my childhood, Murphy had the pleasure of telling me how the Ursuline-run Catholic boarding school she had attended from 1975 to 1979 in Owensboro, Kentucky, had supported and actively participated in the Nestlé boycott. In addition, INFACT itself was actually launched as a branch of the Interfaith Center for Corporate Accountability of the National Council of Churches in the United States. Although the National Council of Churches is the ecumenical body of non-Catholic Christian faith groups in the United States, the man in charge of the Nestlé Boycott campaign, Doug Johnson, was a Vietnam anti-war

activist who had been previously "the director of the Third World Institute located at the Newman Catholic Center." (68)

Johnson had not only been the director of the Newman Center, but he included the centre in the letterhead in the fundraising letter cited at the top of this chapter (Johnson 1979).

INFACT was extremely effective at frame alignment, or "frame bridging" – the bringing together of structurally disconnected and otherwise ideologically unaligned groups to build a collective movement around a common concern (Snow et al. 1986). Another early leaflet listed boycott supporters, including people and organizations as diverse as Ralph Nader, Dr Benjamin Spock, Gloria Steinem, Cesar Chavez, Dr Michael Latham, and several universities, non-profits, and religious institutions (INFACT 1979; Murphy 2012).

Noticeably absent from this list are any primarily Black churches or organizations. Considering the liberal use of images of Black bodies to decry the dangers of formula in "developing countries," the failure to engage with Black organizations is a significant oversight in this coalition building, though consistent with the historical failure to treat Black women as full agents in discussions around breastfeeding. The legacy of racism meant that in the twentieth century, White mothers were depicted as virtuous and good, while Black mothers were depicted as Mammies and Nannies who dote on the White children in their care while ignoring or abusing their own Black babies. Andrea Freeman (2018) argues that the decline in Black American women's breastfeeding rates that began in the 1940s was partly a response to such dehumanizing images:

> In magazines, television, and newspapers the most common image
> of a Black woman nursing, then and now, is not of a nurturing,
> middle-class African American but, instead of a bare-breasted Afri-
> can woman. These types of images, prevalent in the popular maga-
> zine National Geographic and in other "educational" media, make
> breastfeeding by Black women appear to be a primitive practice. This
> is not an image or label with which most Black women in the United
> States want to be associated. (1574)

She goes on to suggest that formula marketing appealed to Black mothers because it was one of the few industries that depicted Black women

Nestlé Boycott Endorsements (Partial List)

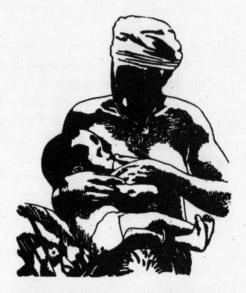

INDIVIDUALS

Dr. Doris Calloway, Chairwoman, Dept. of Nutrition, University of California, Berkeley
Cesar Chavez, President, United Farmworkers
Dick Clark, former U.S. Senator, Iowa
Dr. Elizabeth Hillman, Prof. of Pediatrics, Memorial University, former Secretary, Kenya Ped. Assoc.
Dr. Allan Jackson, Tropical Metabolism Research Unit, Kingston, Jamaica
Dr. Derrick Jelliffe, Head of Division of Population, Family and Public Health, UCLA School of Public Health
Frances Moore Lappe, Author of *Diet for a Small Planet* and *Food First!*
Dr. Michael Latham, Director, Program on International Nutrition, Cornell University
Ralph Nader
Dr. Benjamin Spock
Gloria Steinem

CHURCH ORGANIZATIONS

American Friends Service Committee, Pacific Northwest Region
American Lutheran Church, SE Minnesota and Southern Wisconsin
American Lutheran Church Women
Archdioceses of Roman Catholic Church: San Francisco, St. Paul and Minneapolis; Albany Diocese, Milwaukee Sisters, Denver Justice & Peace, New Orleans Social Apostolate, Rochester NY J & P
Bread for the World (chapters across the country)
Clergy and Laity Concerned
Church Women United
Disciples of Christ Youth Movement
Maryknoll Fathers and Brothers
National Council of Churches
National Association of Women Religious
Presbyterian Church in the U.S.
United Church of Christ (six conferences)
United Methodist Church (twelve conferences, four national offices)

OTHER ORGANIZATIONS

American Medical Student Association
California Nurses Association
College and Student Governments: U.C. Berkeley, Harvard Student Body, U. Penn., Colorado College, Grinnell, Wellesley, Radcliffe, San Jose State, Providence U.
Democratic Parties of Minnesota and Washington State
Institute for Food and Development Policy
Lutheran Student Movement of the U.S.
National Organization for Women (five chapters)
Oxfam-America
Peace Corps volunteers of Cameroon
San Francisco Federation of Teachers
United Farm Workers of America (UFW)
YWCA Cambridge MA, Hartford CT)

NESTLE'S BOYCOTT LIST

Chocolates—
Nestle's CRUNCH; Toll House Chips; Nestle's Quik; Hot Cocoa Mix; Choco'lite; Choco-Bake; $100,000 Candy Bar; Price's Chocolates; Go Ahead Bar

Coffees and Teas—
Taster's Choice; Nescafe; Nestea; Decaf; Sunrise, Pero

Wines—
Beringer Brothers; Los Hermanos; Crosse and Blackwell

Cheeses—
Swiss Knight; Wispride; Gerber Cheeses; Old Fort; Provalone Lacatelli; Cherry Hill; Roger's

Packaged Fruits, Soups, Etc.—
Libby's; Stouffer frozen foods; Souptime; Maggi Soups; Crosse and Blackwell

Hotels and Restaurants—
Stouffer; Rusty Scupper

Miscellaneous—
L'Oreal Cosmetics; Nestle Cookie Mixes; Deer Park Mountain Spring Water; Pine Hill Crystal Water; Kavli Crispbread; McVities; Keiller; James Keller & Son, Ltd.; Contique by Alcon; Ionax by Owen Labs; Lancome

Nestle, a Swiss company, intends to double its U.S. size by 1980 by buying up U.S. companies. This results in many unexpected additions to the Boycott List!

For further information, contact: Infant Formula Action Coalition (INFACT), 1701 University Avenue, SE, Minneapolis, Minnesota 55414. (612) 331-3437.

8.1 a and b (above and opposite) Flyer listing Nestlé boycott endorsements and describing the boycott, 1979.

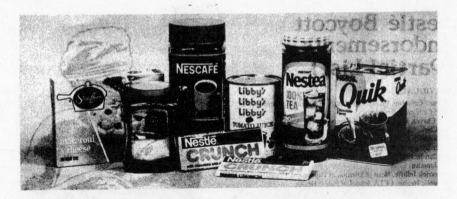

BOYCOTT NESTLÉ

BECAUSE: In Asia, Africa and Latin America, over 10 million babies fed on infant formula suffer "bottle baby disease"—diarrhea, malnutrition, brain damage and even death—every year. Nestle's unethical promotion has made it the world's leading seller of baby formula in developing countries, where misuse is inevitable.

BECAUSE: Since infant formula in poor countries can cost up to 60 percent of the family income, mothers are forced to dilute it—and babies starve. Poor families have too little fuel to sterilize baby bottles, lack refrigerators and have to use contaminated water. The bottle and formula then become carriers of disease. Studies show death rates are 2 to 3 times higher for bottle-fed babies than for breast-fed infants.

BECAUSE: If a woman is convinced to stop breast feeding, within a week her milk can dry up and she is forced to rely on infant formula. Nestle's free samples to mothers (often through doctors) can thus "hook" a mother on formula. Nestle also employs "milk nurses"—saleswomen in medical uniforms—to sell their products to mothers in the hospital. Nestle supplies colorful posters and free medical equipment to hospitals; they give gifts to doctors to enlist their endorsement. In some areas, they <u>continue</u> to advertise through the mass media. Their aggressive promotion has persuaded millions of women to stop breast feeding and use formulas.

BECAUSE: For over eight years nutritionists, doctors and consumer groups have presented reports to Nestle showing that their promotion is contributing to a "bottle baby disaster." Despite these years of mounting criticism—letters, delegations, and even a lawsuit—Nestle has made only the smallest changes in its promotion methods.

BECAUSE: Nestle, a giant food corporation based in Switzerland, wholly owns its U.S. subsidiaries: the Nestle Co., Stouffer, and Libby. The Infant Formula Action Coalition (INFACT), a nationwide coalition of consumer, women's and religious groups, has called a boycott of all Nestle's products until this company stops all promotion which contributes to the "bottle baby disaster."

Speak to Nestle in the language they understand. **BOYCOTT NESTLE!** Write to Pres. David Guerrant, Nestle Company, 100 Bloomingdale Rd., White Plains, NY 10605; tell him why you're Boycotting; expect a reply and ask INFACT for a critique.

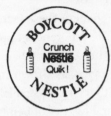

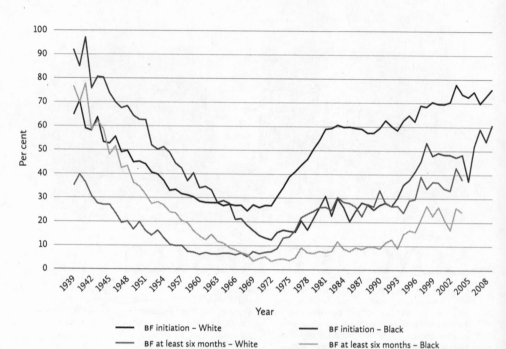

8.2 Rates of breastfeeding initiation and duration of at least six months by Black and White mothers, 1939–2009.

in advertising at all and did so in a positive light. Other explanations for Black women's lower rates of breastfeeding have also included structural racism and poor support within the medical field (Hausman 2003; Freeman 2018), including a lack of Black women as certified lactation consultants (Allers 2017).

Although all of these factors are true, they do not seem to fully explain Black-White differences in breastfeeding rates over time, considering that Black mothers actually had higher rates of breastfeeding from 1939 until the early 1970s, as shown in figure 8.2. If low breastfeeding rates among Black mothers is to be explained by inadequate access to medical supports or a cultural history of being used as wet nurses, why would Black women not have had consistently lower breastfeeding rates than White women since formula first entered the market? While Freeman's (2018) suggestion that formula's positive portrayal of Black women would likely be a compelling carrot to lure them to formula, I can't help but notice that the lagging uptake in Black women's breastfeeding rates coincides with the timing of the Nestlé boycott, an anti-formula campaign led by a White man associated with the Catholic Church and endorsed by a number of primarily White churches, health authorities, and other organizations. To be fair, Cesar Chavez with the United Farm Workers was Mexican American; however, no Black churches or leaders were mentioned in these early documents, despite the liberal usage of Black women's bodies to symbolize victimhood, poverty, and dead babies.

The cover of the 1986 publication of Cicely Williams' "Milk and Murder" speech, discussed in the previous chapter (figure 7.2), depicts a woman with caricatured lips and cans on her breasts, holding what looks like a dead baby up to the skies. Though the image is stylized, it aligns with common racial stereotypes of African women during this era – which is particularly troubling given that the speech was first delivered in Singapore about infant feeding in Singapore, far away from Africa. And though the image of the Black woman breastfeeding on the flyer listing endorsements for the Nestlé boycott (figure 8.1) arguably looks beautiful breastfeeding her baby, she appears to be fully topless. This image was also used as the INFACT organizational logo in its letterhead used to write letters to Congress (ICCR 1979).

Not only were African women's images used to embody victimhood, but the language used by leaders was no better. For example, in the fundraising letter cited in this chapter's epigraph, the national chairperson of INFACT, Douglas A. Johnson, wrote,

> For in places where pure water and knowledge of sterilizing procedures are scarce, artificial milk formula (which, incidentally, lacks natural antibodies found in mother's milk) is like a loaded gun. Improperly prepared, the bottle is a breeding ground for bacteria that cause acute diarrhea, malnutrition and death.
>
> But what chance do these illiterate, impoverished, unsophisticated young women have against the vast resources and subtle advertising techniques of the Nestlé Company and the others? (Johnson 1979, 2)

No wonder Black women may have been less inclined to jump aboard Johnson's anti-formula campaign with him breathlessly begging for someone to just PLEASE think of the Children! Apparently, the poor Black babies need saving from mothers too ignorant to see through the lies of formula hucksters.

Did Anti-formula Campaigns Work?

The Nestlé boycott led to worldwide outcry, and yet restrictions on formula marketing did not increase breastfeeding rates significantly enough to satisfy many international actors. According to Ted Greiner (2000), a well-known scholar and breastfeeding advocate from the Swedish International Development Agency (SIDA), Dr Derrick Jelliffe was frustrated at UNICEF for not moving fast enough to get more babies breastfeeding. However, this changed in 1980 when a new executive director, Jim Grant, took the helm at UNICEF, initiating what he called a "Child Survival and Development Revolution." Part of Grant's revolution involved a new set of healthcare priorities: growth monitoring, oral rehydration therapy, breastfeeding, and immunization (GOBI). This strategy, developed by physician Jon Rohde, later became GOBI-FFF, the Fs standing for food supplementation, family or birth spacing, and female education (Nyi Nyi 2001, 69).

GOBI-FFF was promised to be a low-cost intervention that would "halve child mortality in a decade or two" (Jolly 2001, 50). Years later, Nyi Nyi (2001), one of Grant's former colleagues at UNICEF, reflected that establishing the legitimacy of the program was essential to its ability to spread around the world. In particular, "Legitimation was also conferred by the endorsement of religious leaders. For example, during the promotion of breastfeeding in the Islamic countries, the edict of the world-renowned Al-Azher University of Egypt that the Prophet Mohammad had decreed that all mothers should breastfeed their children for two years dissolved all doubts in the communities of the faithful" (73).

Although religious leaders vocally supported the breastfeeding component of the GOBI strategy, feminists at UNICEF were not so convinced that breastfeeding held the answer to child malnutrition. For instance, Mary Racelis, sociologist and UNICEF senior policy adviser on family and child welfare, voiced support for all but one of the components of the GOBI-FFF strategy:

> The only controversial element among the seven was breastfeeding. Given the ongoing mother versus women struggle, the emphasis on breastfeeding appeared yet again to compartmentalize women

around their maternal roles. Denunciations were rife: were women always to be portrayed in terms of their breasts as the human equivalent of milking cows? Moreover, while breastfeeding was a desirable and natural practice, male advocates like Jim [Grant] had to recognize that it was declining, not because women did not know any better, or not even primarily because the infant formula industry was strongly promoting bottle-feeding. It was declining because women had to work and could not breastfeed even if they wanted to. The prevailing situation in field, factory or market discouraged babies in the workplace, and certainly did not support women's going home to feed them. To the women's network, the breastfeeding campaign ignored the realities of women's lives, compounding that shortsightedness by castigating the victims – women – for turning to bottle-feeding. (2001, 124)

Racelis notes that Grant eventually came to understand the women's arguments, even speaking on the importance of women's empowerment for child survival and health at the UN International Conference on Women in Nairobi, Kenya, in 1985. However, UNICEF remained doggedly focused on increasing rates of exclusive breastfeeding.

In 1990, the WHO released a new policy document, the Innocenti Declaration, developed by a consortium of seventy representatives from thirty countries and major international development organizations including UNICEF, the WHO, the United States Agency for International Development (USAID), and SIDA. Named for the Innocenti Centre in Florence, Italy, where the declaration was signed, the policy sought to address what was seen as a global crisis in breastfeeding. The declaration is a brief document that calls on nations for the "protection, promotion, and support of breastfeeding" and was affirmed by the Forty-Fifth World Health Assembly and by the executive board of UNICEF in 1992 (UNICEF Innocenti Research Centre 2005). According to SIDA's Ted Greiner, there were four primary reasons that this document was necessary:

1 It contained important language for breastfeeding promotion, particularly the following: "all women should be enabled to practice exclusive breastfeeding and infants should be fed exclusively on breast milk from birth to 4–6 months of age. Thereafter, children should continue to be breastfed, while receiving appropriate

complementary foods, for up to two years of age or beyond"
[Innocenti Declaration].

2 It came up with four operational targets that governments should
   strive to attain. They included (a) appointing a national breastfeeding coordinator of appropriate authority and a national
   breastfeeding committee, (b) ensuring that every maternity facility
   practiced the Ten Steps to Successful Breastfeeding, (c) taking
   action to give effect to the International Code, and (d) enacting
   legislation to protect the breastfeeding rights of working women.

3 The language used in this final point introduced the concept of
   breastfeeding being a human right.

4 It attempted to involve high-level participants from a large and
   representative group of countries, both developing and industrial-
   ized. (Greiner 2000, 2)

According to Greiner (2000), Latin American countries opposed recom-
mending this time frame, saying that six months was enough, but delegates from predominantly Muslim countries refused to support anything
less than two years on the basis that this length of time is recommended in
the Qur'an. Despite religious origins, six months of exclusive breastfeeding
and two years of non-exclusive breastfeeding is the definitive *health* recommendation given to new mothers around the world, including by the
WHO (2020) and the Public Health Agency of Canada (2021). However, the
US CDC (2020) uses the American Academy of Pediatrics recommendation
of six months of exclusive breastfeeding "and then gradually adding solid
foods while continuing breastfeeding until at least the baby's first birthday.
Thereafter, breastfeeding can be continued for as long as both mother and
baby desire it" (AAP 2014).

Prior to this time, not only was there no consensus as to two years
of breastfeeding, but the idea of two years was seen as absurd by some
within breastfeeding advocacy. For example, in response to a statement
that Nestlé distributed to the Governing Board of the National Council of
Churches (an organization active in the Nestlé boycott), INFACT suggested
that such a recommendation was a straw man created by Nestlé to make
breastfeeding advocates sound ridiculous. They criticize Nestlé's statement that formula supplementation at three months has been shown to be
useful in developing countries among malnourished mothers noting that

The 3-month "crisis" is based on one study in West Africa, and contradicts a number of surveys that demonstrate that mother's milk is
usually sufficient for the first 5 or 6 months. But, of course, at some
point mother's milk must be supplemented with other foods. It is
ridiculous and another of Nestlé's "strawman" arguments to suggest
their critics support exclusive breast-feeding for two years! (ICCR,
Infant Formula Program 1979)

Soon after the Innocenti Declaration, in 1991 the WHO and UNICEF
launched the Baby-friendly Hospital Initiative (BFHI) to encourage hospitals to support breastfeeding and curtail formula marketing in medical
settings, despite the anger this aroused in feminists at the UN for failing
to take into account the realities of women's lives (Racelis 2001). Recently
updated, the BFHI aims "to implement the Ten Steps to Successful Breastfeeding and to end the distribution of free and low-cost supplies of breast-
milk substitutes to health facilities" (WHO and UNICEF n.d.). The "Ten
Steps" are divided into management procedures and clinical practices (and
seem to have employed multiple subpoints for step one in the recent up-
dates, perhaps to avoid changing the name to the "twelve steps"):

Critical management procedures:
1a Comply fully with the *International Code of Marketing of Breast-
    milk Substitutes* and relevant World Health Assembly resolutions.
1b Have a written infant feeding policy that is routinely communi-
    cated to staff and parents.
1c Establish ongoing monitoring and data-management systems.
2   Ensure that staff have sufficient knowledge, competence and
    skills to support breastfeeding.

Key clinical practices:
3   Discuss the importance and management of breastfeeding with
    pregnant women and their families.
4   Facilitate immediate and uninterrupted skin-to-skin contact
    and support mothers to initiate breastfeeding as soon as possible
    after birth.
5   Support mothers to initiate and maintain breastfeeding and
    manage common difficulties.

6   Do not provide breastfed newborns any food or fluids other than breast milk, unless medically indicated.
7   Enable mothers and their infants to remain together and to practise rooming-in 24 hours a day.
8   Support mothers to recognize and respond to their infants' cues for feeding.
9   Counsel mothers on the use and risks of feeding bottles, teats and pacifiers.
10   Coordinate discharge so that parents and their infants have timely access to ongoing support and care. (WHO and UNICEF n.d.)

To be a designated a "baby-friendly" hospital, its maternity staff must take courses and facilities must undertake self-appraisals and external assessments. One could summarize the BFHI as supporting the creation of conditions where mothers would be pushed in the direction of breast-feeding through the "carrot" of increased support and the "stick" of banning alternatives to breast milk. According to the BFHI website, "Since its launching BFHI has grown, with more than 152 countries around the world implementing the initiative" (WHO 2018). Public awareness of the initiative received a boost in 2012, when then New York City mayor Michael Bloomberg launched the "Latch On NYC" campaign "urging hospitals to stop giveaways and monitor formula like other medical supplies, stored in locked cabinets and accounted for when mothers have medical needs or request it," to which "28 of 40 hospitals have agreed" (Belluck 2012).

Although there has been significant uptake in BFHI accreditation, actual implementation and results are unclear. In their report to the Agency for Healthcare Research and Quality within the US Department of Health and Human Services, Cynthia Feltner et al. (2018) reviewed the strength of the evidence for a number of breastfeeding programs and policies. They found "moderate" evidence that BFHI improved rates of breastfeeding duration, but evidence was "low" that it improved rates of initiation. Nonetheless, the authors expressed support for the BFHI as an effective program.

Fallon, Harrold, and Chisholm (2019) came to less favourable conclusions of BFHI in the United Kingdom, identifying very few quality studies linking its implementation with breastfeeding outcomes, and zero studies on its impact on other maternal or infant health outcomes. They concluded that there is very little quantitative evidence that BFHI positively affects breastfeeding outcomes and that any effects that can be identified are of very short duration (i.e. the first seven days). Additionally, in their review of qualitative evidence, they found that although healthcare providers can be highly influential in getting more women to breastfeed, BFHI may "promote unrealistic expectations of breastfeeding, not meet women's individual needs, and foster negative emotional experiences" (20).

Not only are there gaps in evidence for its effectiveness, but it is unclear to what degree the BFHI is being implemented, even in hospitals achieving BFHI designation (Nelson and Grossniklaus 2019; Zarshenas et al. 2018). For example, Jennifer Nelson and Daurice Grossniklaus (2019) analyzed maternity practices in infant nutrition and care (mPINC) data collected by the CDC, finding that although aspects of BFHI had been adopted between 2009 and 2014, the initiative had a relatively limited impact on hospital-wide breastfeeding policies. Specifically, whereas maternity wards tend to have clear breastfeeding policies, other units like radiology or the emergency room may lack procedures for supporting breastfeeding (Nelson and Grossniklaus 2019). Although the authors did not call attention to this, my reading of their findings suggests that hospitals were most likely to implement the recommendations that would save them money. For instance, hospitals that implemented some of the BFHI recommendations were more likely to eliminate or limit free formula (14.1 per cent increase) or pacifiers (21 per cent increase) but less likely to begin assessing staff competency (6 per cent increase) or offer more prenatal breastfeeding education (7.8 per cent increase) (Nelson and Grossniklaus 2019). Along these lines, the authors did reference a study that found higher rates of exclusive breastfeeding in hospitals that paid "fair market value for infant formula" (Bai et al. 2016, 5).

Despite such questions about the effectiveness of breastfeeding promotion in addressing issues rooted in poverty, in 2012 the non-governmental organization Save the Children issued a report entitled *Superfood for Babies: How Overcoming Barriers to Breastfeeding Will Save Children's Lives* (Mason, Rawe, and Wright 2013). The document draws on much of the same language and arguments made by the WHO, UNICEF, and other health agencies and NGOs. Among those the authors thank for contributing to the report is the UK branch of IBFAN – an organization focused on implementing the International Code of Marketing of Breast-milk Substitutes fully around the world. *Superfood for Babies* is full of easily tweetable and shocking statistics, including the claim that 6.9 million children under age five died in 2011 and that "830,000 newborn deaths could be prevented every year if all infants were given breast milk in the first hour of life." They go on to write, "Breastfeeding saves lives. It's the closest thing there is to a 'silver bullet' in the fight against malnutrition and newborn deaths" (vii).

In a discourse analysis of this document, Watson and Mason point out that this "language of risk – typical of neoliberal public health campaigns and development projects alike – decontextualizes maternal and infant health in deceptive ways, placing the onus, once again, squarely on the shoulders of women in the most precarious of circumstances" (2015, 575). Focusing resources on breastfeeding as a solution to the impact of global poverty has become a standard global-development strategy. As I will discuss in the next chapter, few countries have taken this as seriously as Indonesia.

9 Saving the Children of Indonesia

Article 128

(1) Every child has the right to receive breast milk exclusively from birth for a minimum of 6 (six) months, unless there is a medical indication to the contrary.

(2) During the breastfeeding period, the family, the Government, the Local Government and the community must give full support to the mother's infant by providing time and special facilities.

(3) Provision of specialised facilities as referred to in paragraph (2) shall be implemented in the workplace and in public facilities.

Article 129

(1) The Government shall be responsible for stipulating policies in order to guarantee the rights of infants to be exclusively breastfed.

(2) Further provisions as referred to in paragraph (1) shall be governed by Government Regulations.

Article 200

Any person who intentionally hinders exclusive breastfeeding programmes as referred to in Article 128 paragraph (2) shall be sentenced to a term of imprisonment (maximum 1 year) and/or to a fine (maximum amount of Rp. 100,000,000.00; One hundred million Rupiah)

Article 201 (1)

(1) In the case that criminal acts are committed by a corporation as referred to in Article 190 paragraph (1), Article 191, Article 192, Article 196, Article 197, Article 198, Article 199, and/or Article 200, in addition to imprisonment and fines against management, a penalty can be imposed on the corporation in the form of a fine, 3 (three) times as severe as the fine referred to in Article 190 paragraph (1), Article 191, Article 192, Article 196, Article 197, Article 198, Article 199 and Article 200.

(2) In addition to criminal penalties as described in paragraph (1), the corporation may also be penalised in the form of a:
    a. Revocation of business permit; and/or
    b. Revocation of status as a legal entity.

Health Law No. 36/2009,
"Law and Regulations on Breastfeeding," Indonesia

Although my research had focused primarily on the United States and Canada, I became interested in breastfeeding promotion in Indonesia following that country's decision to make breastfeeding mandatory for at least six months. In the fall of 2018, I travelled to Indonesia to learn more about what had led to the mandatory breastfeeding law. Through contacts with faculty at Gadjah Mada University in Yogyakarta, I was matched up with an unbelievably helpful anthropology graduate student and part-time worker for a local health authority, Endang Purwasari, who served as my translator and research assistant in the field. Endang and I became fast friends, laughing at my cultural faux pas as we moved through the streets of Jakarta and Yogyakarta talking with mothers and leaders of various national and international agencies. Endang also took me to different grocery stores to peruse the formula offerings and led me on cultural tours of various landmarks, giving me a crash course in Indonesian history and culture. Though I still would not consider myself an expert, I learned an immense amount about a culture that I had known very little about before I began researching breastfeeding. Through my field work there, as I tried to come to grips with why the law came to pass and what it meant for everyday women, I stumbled upon a mystery involving formula company involvement in the creation of the law that has likely led to increased profits in the company's non-formula holdings, to the detriment of the Indonesian people.

A Crash Course on Indonesia

In her 2009 book, *Gender, Islam, and Democracy in Indonesia*, Kathryn Robinson explains how "traditional" gender roles were constructed in this diverse Southeast Asian archipelago made up of people speaking hundreds of languages, with differing customs and religions (now primarily Islam). Traditionally, there were areas of Indonesia where gender was not firmly related to sex, where matrilineal descent led women to have more local power, and where language emphasized generation over gender. Among wealthier Indonesians, as part of the anticolonial movement in the early twentieth century, there were also a number of feminist groups that formed to fight for women's rights to education and against polygamy.

It was only with the rise of the authoritarian, militaristic leader Suharto in the late 1960s that the gender roles Westerners think of as "traditional" were invented and enforced through a series of government-mandated agencies and laws. Suharto's dictatorial reign began with the slaughter of over a million Indonesians; bolstered by the United States, he remained in power until 1998 (Vltchek 2012). Suharto used gender to unite the country's ethnically and religiously diverse groups, promoting a belief in men's and women's proper roles and promising men that they were entitled to "sexual and domestic service from their wives" (K. Robinson 2009, 87). Within this government, the wives of male civil servants were required to serve in state agencies that taught women to accept this subordinate and home-focused role. Since then, women have challenged and succeeded in dismantling many of these policies, but Suharto's tenure coincided with neoliberal global trends and a parallel rise of Islam in Indonesian politics, resulting in the country's current status as a liberal economy with a patriarchal, gendered division of labour. Specifically, Suharto's anti-communist "New Order" government liberalized the Indonesian economy by opening trade with Western countries. Although this initially invigorated the economy, widespread corruption and broader economic instability caused the Indonesian economy to be hard hit by the Asian financial crisis of the late 1990s. The brutality of Suharto's regime eventually came to an end when he was overthrown in 1998.

During the period that followed, known as the Reformasi (Reformation) period, international actors took greater control of the country's economic and political decision-making. In particular, the International Monetary Fund predicated its bailouts on increased access to the island nation by multinational corporations. Western actors, including Bill and Hillary Clinton, hailed Indonesia as a shining star of global development, but scholar Andre Vltchek (2012) has shown that corruption remained rampant. Today, the country's economy continues to rely on resource extraction by external actors rather than building its own capacity for industrial development.

In the Field

By the end of the trip Endang and I had conducted eighteen formal interviews with twenty women. We spoke with three representatives from the national breastfeeding support group AIMI-ASI (a director at the national office in Jakarta and two volunteers in Yogyakarta) and representatives from the Indonesian office of the WHO, UN Women, and a national women's advocacy organization. We also spoke to the head of a *Posyandu* (a local healthcare centre) and more than ten Indonesian mothers who had recently given birth. I was often stopped randomly by people on the street who asked to take their picture with me as if I were a celebrity, and whenever they had a baby with them, I asked Endang to find out if they had breastfed their child. She would often laugh, somewhat embarrassed to pry into the private lives of strangers, but in the name of research she courageously made the inquiry of all the women. They always said they breastfed exclusively.

The mothers I formally interviewed came from different socioeconomic classes and included labourers, seamstresses, teachers, housewives (one on a livestock farm), graduate students, entrepreneurs, and professional women working in skyscrapers in the capital city. All of the women were married, and of those who disclosed their religious affiliation most were Muslim, but two or three were Christian. Most of the agency representatives were also mothers and all but three of the women whom we spoke to about their own feeding experiences said they exclusively breastfed. Only two mothers admitted to formula feeding for any extended period, one of whom was sampled as an agency representative, so her daughter was an older child at the time of the interview. A third mother fed her child formula for just two days and then went on to breastfeed exclusively. Because Endang worked for the *Posyandu*, she suggested that some women might tell us they exclusively breastfed out of a desire to appear to be following the rules. She suggested this might explain why one woman we had been referred to as a possible formula feeder stated that no, she had only breastfed for the required six months.

Many of the women had their babies with them during the interviews, and all the babies were adorable. Except for the White European representative of UN Women, all the other women we spoke to were Indonesian nationals. Interviews were conducted sometimes in English, sometimes in Bahasa Indonesian, and sometimes in a mix of both. Endang would run the interviews when in Bahasa Indonesian but fill me in periodically to give the summary of what they were talking about. After a while, I started to pick up a few words: ASI (breast milk), *eksklusif* (exclusive), *air* (water), *susu formula* (formula).

During my inquiry into what had gone into the law mandating breastfeeding, representatives from both the WHO and AIMI-ASI mentioned the name Utami Roesli, crediting her as a key leader in breastfeeding promotion in Indonesia. Roesli is a board-certified pediatrician, fellow of the Academy of Breastfeeding Medicine, an international board-certified lactation consultant (IBCLC), and co-founder of the Indonesian Breast-feeding Center (Wise 2011). Given her position as an international breast-feeding advocate, prior to my trip I had assumed that Roesli was one of the primary drivers of the law that made breastfeeding mandatory for all mothers. I had read her quoted in a PBS NewsHour article as saying, "The information that mothers get here in Indonesia about breastfeeding is very, very little compared to what they get about formula because the formula companies are so powerful ... [T]his law tips the scales back to breastfeeding" (Wise 2011).

However, a leader of AIMI-ASI adamantly disputed that Roesli and other breastfeeding supporters had wanted a law *requiring* breastfeeding. Rather, they had wanted more support in place for mothers who want to breastfeed and wanted to block undue influence from formula companies. As this leader shared with us, in reference to the law,

It's not that bad, but there are some things that are missing and it's very concerning for us. Because the first thing is they oblige: every mother should breastfeed. I said, why we have to? Everyone should support us. The doctor should support us. The midwives should support us. The family members. Not the mother! It is very concerning for us to read that, that way, as if we are very stupid and we don't understand.

From the perspective of AIMI-ASI, laws should protect mothers from those who would put obstacles in the way of breastfeeding – the burden should not be foisted on mothers alone.

In addition to providing direct support to mothers, AIMI-ASI has focused heavily on stopping the marketing and promotion of formula. Although it is a grassroots group of Indonesian women, it has partnered with and been supported by a number of outside organizations and individuals, including Canadian breastfeeding advocate Dr Jack Newman, founder of the International Breastfeeding Centre in Toronto; Dr Elisabeth Sterken of INFACT Canada and IBFAN North America; and the International Baby Foods Action Network (IBFAN). IBFAN describes itself as a watchdog organization whose mission is to protect breastfeeding through the monitoring of "baby food corporations' misleading propaganda, advocating with governments to hold the baby food corporations accountable, providing technical and planning support to governments, campaigning, training and capacity building" ("Our Mission" 2018, n.p.). With support from these organizations, AIMI-ASI was working on drafting legislation to increase the regulations on labelling infant formula and prohibiting companies from marketing it to children under thirty-six months – lengthening this prohibition from its current minimum age of twelve months. Among AIMI-ASI's concerns are the poor state of sanitation in Indonesia and an incident in which poisoned formula failed to be recalled.

As the story of the law was told to me by a leader of AIMI-ASI, around 2007 the Indonesian government invited AIMI-ASI, along with representatives from the Ministry of Health, the Ministry of Trade, and formula companies, to participate in drafting new legislation regarding infant feeding. As AIMI-ASI tried to push for greater controls over corporations, the formula companies and trade ministry officials pushed back, arguing that any limits on formula milk would have a detrimental impact on the national economy. The AIMI-ASI leaders were disbelieving of this as a real concern, given that there is little dairy production within their island nation and most milk is imported. As the legislators made their final version of the law, the breastfeeding advocates were dis-invited. Rumour had it that the law was written "over lunch with the formula company," though I have no evidence to prove this.

The breastfeeding mandate, printed in full at the start of this chapter, was one small part of a larger piece of legislation, Health Law 36, enacted in 2009 to replace a 1992 health policy, Health Law 23. Health Law 36 covers a range of issues including health service facilities, emergency health response, medical supply management, health technology development and distribution, patient protections, disease prevention and recovery, and reproductive health including banning abortion except in cases of rape or risk to mother or fetus. While Indonesian breastfeeding advocates were looped out of the law's development, international agencies had been looped in. According to remarks written in English and appended to the law by the Indonesian Parliament Forum for Population and Development, the law was translated into English as to reflect collaboration with the United Nations Population Fund (UNFPA), the UN's sexual and reproductive health agency. In keeping with the goals of international health agencies, Health Law 36 was followed by policies enacted in 2012 and 2013 that explicitly include the WHO's Baby-friendly Hospital Initiative's "Ten Steps to Successful Breastfeeding."

Under Article 200 of Health Law 36, the penalty for interfering with mothers' ability to exclusively breastfeed is a fine of 100,000,000 rupiah and possible imprisonment of up to one year. According to the Indonesian Statistical Agency, the mean monthly income in February 2016 was 2,180,577 rupiah (BPS 2017), meaning that this fine is about four times higher than the average annual income of Indonesians. Given that the law asserts the infant's "right to receive exclusive breastfeeding for 6 months," one might worry about the penalty for mothers who do not breastfeed; however, in a news interview, Dr Minarto, director of nutrition for the Indonesian Ministry of Health, stated that "the government does not intend to lock up mothers who don't breastfeed ... [T]his law is intended to provide support to them" (Wise 2011).

The nature of this "support" wasn't defined until three years after the initial law was passed. In 2012 the government issued Policy No. 33, "On the Exclusive Breastfeeding," which required lactation rooms in workplaces and public areas (such as health service facilities, hotels, airports, and shopping centres) where health information about the benefits of breastfeeding would be displayed. The policy further states that "the organizer of public areas such as health services facilities have to support the success of exclusive breastfeeding program referring to the following 10 (ten) steps towards the successful attainment in breastfeeding" (Indonesia 2012, chap. 5, Art. 33), which are basically identical to the BFHI ten steps. For their part, national and provincial governments were made legally responsible for breastfeeding advocacy, policy, research, and technology and for integrating breastfeeding into health service curricula, providing staff to counsel women about breastfeeding, and ensuring access to information and education about breastfeeding.

According to Policy No. 33, "supporting mothers to breastfeed" means that healthcare providers may not provide formula to infants, with a few exceptions. The exact situations in which babies may be deprived of their "right to be exclusively breastfed" are strictly defined by the 2013 Policy No. 39, "On Infant Formula Milk and Other Baby Products," as follows:

1. Every mother who gives birth has to give exclusive breastfeeding for infants ... except in the circumstances of:
   a. medical indications;
   b. mother does not exist, or
   c. the mother is separated from the baby.

2. In the circumstances referred to in paragraph (1), mother, family, medical personnel and other health staff can provide Infant Milk Formula. (Indonesia, Ministry of Health 2013, chap. 3, pt. 1, Art. 6)

Medical indications must be determined by a doctor (though a midwife or nurse is allowed if a doctor is unavailable) and must fall within a list of serious infant health conditions including extremely low birth weight (under 1,500 grams), a rare genetic condition called maple syrup urine disease (MSUD), galactosemia, phenylketonuria, and other metabolic abnormalities. In some of these cases, such as phenylketonuria, a disorder in which ingestion of too much protein and certain chemicals can lead to brain damage, breastfeeding is still encouraged under the "supervision of a competent pediatrician" (chap. 3, pt. 1, para. 2, Art. 8[3]). Mothers can also be exempted if they have HIV, have herpes simplex virus (HSV-1 or HSV-2) in the breast, or are taking particular medications, such as Iodine-131 radioactive or chemotherapy cytotoxic (Art. 12). The policy also describes proper procedure for the use of formula in emergency and/or disaster situations, where the mother's or donor milk might be unavailable.

The marketing of formula is also highly circumscribed under this policy; particular prescriptions and proscriptions related to language include the following: "Advertisement material ... shall contain a statement that the Infant Formula Milk can only be granted on certain conditions as set forth in Article 6, as well as information that Breast Milk is the best food for babies" (Indonesia, Ministry of Health 2013, chap. 5, pt. 1, Art. 20[2]). Any advertising also must get special permission from the minister prior to printing, and the following long list of marketing strategies are prohibited:

a   providing of products sample free of charge;
b   provision of free supply, rebates, or any form of the purchase of Infant Formula Milk as [an] attraction [to] the seller;
c   providing awards for those who [are] able to sell and/or purchase Infant Formula Milk;
d   sell or offer by exaggerating products via telephone, email and other electronic means;
e   offer or sale of Infant Formula Milk directly using either a sales marketing services that come to your home or place of public facilities;

f use of health staff to provide information about the Infant Formula Milk to the public;

g using healthy baby picture that seems to be healthy because of the
use of its products; and

h idealize the product as if it was the best. (chap. 5, pt. 2, Art. 21)

The penalty for companies that violate the law is "(a) verbal reprimand,
and/or; (b) written reprimand," whereas health staff can be sanctioned by
"(a) verbal warning; (b) written reprimand, and/or (c) revocation of license"
(chap. 10, Art. 30[1][2]).

Given the history of unethical formula marketing in Indonesia, I can
see legitimate reasons for restricting the activities of formula producers.
Journalist Zoe Williams (2013) wrote a compelling article in the *Guardian*
detailing the tactics these companies used to try to get more babies on the
bottle. For instance, Danone subsidiary Sari Husada set up contracts with
Indonesian midwives that rewarded them based on the number of formula
boxes they sold in a month. Danone says that it has replaced this payment
system with training for midwives, but a former worker quoted in the
article stated that in 2012 the company shifted from paying cash commis-
sions to paying with gifts in kind. Williams writes, "The spokesperson for
Danone insists that ... the gifts are just that, an act of beneficence to the
midwife, to help her set up her practice, they are unconditional upon the
sales of any formula." Gifts notably include items such as televisions, lap-
tops, and actual medical supplies like "an oxygen canister, a TENS machine
or a nebuliser" (n.p.).

One marketing technique that I struggled to believe until I saw it with
my own eyes was that of paying women to stand in grocery stores to offer
information to prospective buyers. Representatives of the companies can
be found in the formula aisles, wearing professional-looking outfits that
are colour coordinated to their brand, holding a clipboard and ready to
offer information about formula for anyone over six months old. They are
able to get around the anti-marketing law in part because in Indonesia, it
is possible to purchase formula not just for babies but for every age group.
There are powdered milks for pregnant women, toddlers, older children,
adults, and older populations, each with a shining face on the box promising better nutrition to those who consume it. This means that although
the Indonesian formula market has been estimated to be worth $1.1 billion,

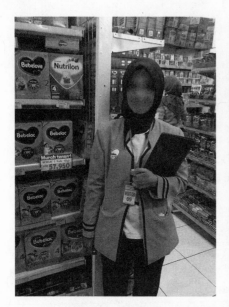 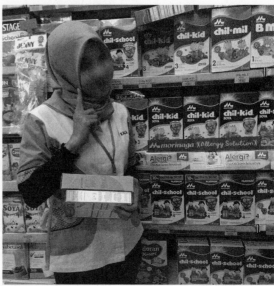

9.1 a and b Representatives from formula companies offering in-store marketing.

this figure may include formulas targeted to populations not covered by the anti-marketing policies. Rather clever.

In my interview with a founder of AIMI-ASI, I kept pressing a question that truly puzzled me: If formula makers were at the table writing legislation to promote breastfeeding as early as 2007, and the 2009 law was purportedly finalized over a lunch between political leaders and formula execs, what possible profit or benefit would the formula companies be seeking to pursue? Her theory was that as the grassroots breastfeeding movement grew and became more influential, the government felt pressured to respond with something and therefore made a law that was toothless. In fact, AIMI-ASI tried to bring forward a test case to apply the law but the organization was unable to come up with a way to use the law to demand any accountability from formula companies. The only case it could make was that of doctors or midwives violating the law, but it was not interested in creating enemies with the medical providers whom AIMI-ASI wanted on its side. The law was most definitely useless in terms of being able to bring charges in court.

Still, Endang and I both pressed the issue with the AIMI-ASI representative, asking why formula manufacturers would actively support a law stating that "every baby is entitled to a mother's milk exclusively from birth

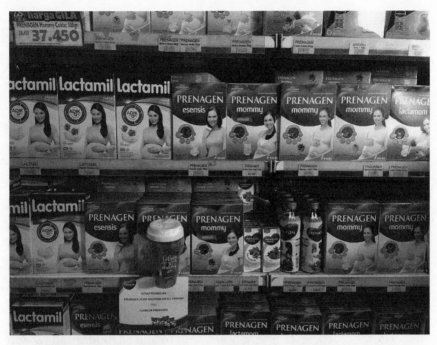

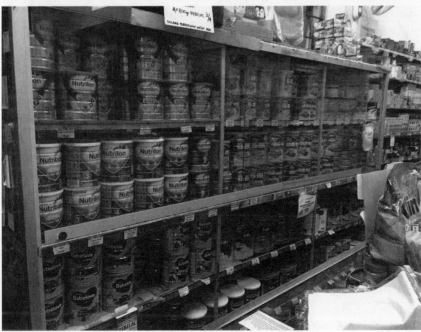

9.2 a and b Shelves of infant formula fill grocery store aisles.

for 6 (six) months, except for medical indications." Why would they want to prohibit their own product, especially given that AIMI-ASI did not want breastfeeding to become a legal requirement for women? In the end, all she could answer was "I don't know." We left the meeting still puzzled by why a mandatory breastfeeding law would emerge from a table of formula manufacturers and politicians who purportedly didn't really care about breastfeeding. I became obsessed with solving this mystery and the answer came to me after a particularly bad case of diarrhea.

There's No Such Thing as a Formula Company

Barely making it through the end of the interview, I found myself doubled over with stomach pains. I had just survived a sleepless night in the bathroom after accidentally licking tap water from my hands after dipping them in a finger bowl in a Jakarta restaurant the night before my interview with the AIMI-ASI representative. We left the interview and arrived at the hotel just in time for me to make it to the blessed bathroom I so desperately needed. Endang kindly went out to find an Indonesian version of saltines and bottled water for me, and I lay in bed hoping the pain would go away. As I lay there, the realization overcame me that no mother would ever knowingly give her baby untreated tap water in Jakarta or anywhere else with similarly poor water quality. Explosive diarrhea is more instructive than the best teacher at the finest educational institution anywhere – and this is not a lesson one needs to learn twice. As I stared vacantly at the mountain of water bottles Endang and I had been drinking and using to brush our teeth, I noticed that most of them said Danone and a number said Nestlé. "Huh," I thought to myself, "those are the same companies that make the most popular brands of formula here."

Later that day, Endang and I flew to Yogyakarta and I began piecing together a theory as I looked through the annual reports of Nestlé and Danone. What I immediately discovered is that there is no such thing as a formula company. Rather, there are multinational corporations that make formula as one branch of their shareholdings, and the two biggest multinationals – Nestlé and Danone – also make bottled water. I mentioned this to my husband, Joel, that night over the phone and he responded with an illuminating story. In the early 2000s, Joel had worked for a marketing company contracted by a food and beverage company to help it rebrand its water division in light of negative media coverage of how plastic water bottles are bad for the environment. Whereas in the 1970s bottled water was associated with health and highbrow consumption (think Evian or Perrier), there had been a shift, and people weren't seeing bottled water the same way. According to Joel, the water executive told him "there's a train coming right at us and we need you to help us stop it." I hung up realizing that mandatory breastfeeding may have helped to stop that train.

Indonesia's Water Problem

The two largest manufacturers of formula globally are Switzerland-based Nestlé and France-based Danone. Nestlé was founded in 1866 as a canned milk company by German-born pharmacist Henri Nestlé, who brought his first infant formula to market in 1867. According to the Nestlé website, that first formula combined "cow's milk, wheat flour and sugar [developed] for consumption by infants who cannot be breastfed, to tackle high mortality rates." Nestlé entered the water market later, with the acquisition of French water bottler Vittel in 1969, followed by France's Perrier Group in 1992 and then Italian mineral water bottler Sanpellegrino Group in 1998 – the same year it launched Nestlé Pure Life "in developing countries, to guarantee clean and healthy drinking water" (Nestlé n.d.). In 2002, it renamed its separate water business "Nestlé Waters" and focused its ambitions on "nutrition, health, and wellness," setting its sights on expanding "in the US, Eastern Europe and Asia, [with] targets for global leadership in water, ice cream and animal food." By 2006, Nestlé developed a "creating shared value approach to business," focusing on "sustainable supply chains in cocoa and coffee while strengthening its position in traditional segments, infant formula and frozen food ... [and] medical nutrition" (Nestlé n.d.).

Like Nestlé, Danone markets itself as a company on a mission to save the world's children, but Danone originally sought to save Spanish children from intestinal infections by introducing yogurt to Barcelona in 1919. It eventually purchased Evian in 1970 along with other food producers, "becoming France's largest producer of beverages and baby food" ("Our Epic History" 2021). Like Nestlé, Danone went on to develop a "new vision of corporate social responsibility" with a "ground-breaking speech" to its executives by then president Antoine Riboud. By the 1990s, it had expanded its food holdings, acquiring the water company Volvic and spreading internationally by targeting Asia in 1991 with a Hong Kong–based food company. In 2007, the same year the Indonesian government invited AIMI-ASI to develop a breastfeeding law, Danone purchased Royal Numico, for $16.8 billion, "to forge what it said will be the world's largest health and nutrition company" (Michelson and Stevenson 2007). In a YouTube video accompanying this piece of its historical legacy, the company notes that "Danone is now world number 2 in water and world number 1 in fresh dairy products." The video ends with the statement that "Numico's international presence on the infant nutrition and medical nutrition market offers Danone a new lever for growth, profitability, and expansion towards emerging countries, particularly in Asia" (Danone 2018).

The annual reports of Danone and Nestlé tell a story of how the "runaway train" of anti-water environmental advocacy may have been slowed down. As bottled water profits declined in western Europe, they needed to find a new market. In its 2007 financial statement, Nestlé Waters Home and Office Delivery in Europe stated that "the unfavourable evolution of the business in various countries, notably in the United Kingdom, together with the increase in interest rates since the beginning of the year have indicated signs of impairment" (Nestlé 2008). In part, the company's financial struggles were likely driven by anti–bottled water activism. As Tony Clarke describes in *Inside the Bottle*,

During the course of 2005, bottled water started to emerge as an issue for education and action in several sectors of society. Consumer groups began to look at the price gouging that goes on in the bottled water industry. Health activists started to focus attention on the chemical and bacteriological contaminants in bottled water. Environmental networks began to address the greenhouse gas emissions and chemical leaching associated with the use of plastic bottles. And, in some instances, poor urban communities started to see how bottled water creates a new rich-poor divide in terms of water as a human right.

At the same time, public sector unions began to actively defend water services by questioning the promotion of bottled water in places. In schools, colleges, and universities, student groups started to openly challenge the exclusivity contracts signed between their administrations and major corporate players in the bottled water industry. And many faith-based communities began to focus public attention on the ethics of bottled water as a prime example of the commodification of the building blocks of life itself on this planet. (2007, 7–8)

As water sales stagnated in Europe, Southeast Asia must have looked like a land of business opportunity, given widespread drinking water problems, shaky economies, and cheap currencies. Investing in the Asian market yielded results: between 1996 and 2006, the Asian share of Danone's holdings more than doubled, from 7 per cent to 17 per cent. By 2008, Asia-Pacific Indonesia made up over 45 per cent of Danone's business, and the firm's subsidiary Aqua had become "number one in Indonesia with over 50% of the market and first worldwide by volume with annual sales topping 6 billion liters" (Danone 2009, 74). Thomas Kunz, executive vice president (Waters), wrote in Danone's 2008 annual report,

In 2008, there was a gap between emerging markets, with growth of nearly 15%, and mature markets in Western Europe, which held steady or lost ground. Our local brands in Mexico, Argentina, Indonesia and China thus posted outstanding growth, while Volvic and Evian ran into headwinds in the UK, Spain and France.

Bottled waters had to contend with increased competition from sweetened beverages and sodas, as well as reduced consumer purchasing power and questions about our environmental impact. We responded energetically with a communications campaign stressing the unique character and benefits of our waters, and also stepped up our environmental responsibility initiatives. We are now making bottles with 25% recycled PET, and Evian is moving toward carbon neutrality ... Finally, we have taken steps to control costs and strengthen our health positioning, and *we are expanding our product ranges and distribution networks, focusing particularly on increasing away-from-home consumption* [my italics] and more effective use of neighborhood sales channels. Against this backdrop, we are heading into 2009 with determination in the tough markets, *and enthusiasm in emerging markets* [my italics]. (Danone 2009, 24)

Danone's enthusiasm in Indonesia was warranted, as evidenced by a 2016 article the company posted to the website Medium, which noted, "with more than 14,000 employees and 21 plants, Indonesia is one of Danone's biggest markets" (Danone 2016, n.p.). This same report links the company's interests in water and infant feeding, specifically through growth in Indonesia:

> Danone settled in Indonesia in 1998 by signing a strategic alliance with Aqua, an Indonesian brand of bottled water launched in 1973. With this partnership, the brand strengthened its market position becoming the largest producer of bottled mineral water in Indonesia ... Danone implemented its Baby Nutrition division in Indonesia in 2007, with the acquisition of Numico and therefore of the brands Sari Husada (an Indonesian brand born in 1954) and PT NIS (launched in Indonesia in 1987 thanks to the import of products from Netherlands). With the launch of SGM in 1965, Sari Husada was a pioneer in the development of production of infant formula in Indonesia ...
>
> With China, Indonesia forms a bridgehead for our growth in the Asia-Pacific region. Thanks to our Aqua and Mizone brands, we occupy the top spot in the Indonesian waters market.
>
> But we're leaders in early life nutrition as well, with our SGM and Sari Husada brands holding 40% of the market. Sales of these two categories alone come to over €1 billion, and Aqua's total volume of bottled water is the largest distributed by Danone anywhere in the world.
>
> Over the past decade, economic growth has halved the number of Indonesians living in extreme poverty, but malnutrition, climate change and natural disasters are a threat to food safety and better nutrition for all. Against this backdrop, providing healthy, affordable food and beverages for as many people as possible is a daily challenge but we're working to meet it by creating an offer that meets local needs.
>
> By pursuing these efforts in close partnership with local associations, health professionals and communities, we're solidifying Danone's positions and promoting sustainable growth in Indonesia. (Danone 2016, n.p.)

While both Danone and Nestlé have sought to position themselves as altruistic stewards of environmental responsibility and health, they, along with other bottled water companies, nonetheless profit where access to clean water is scarce. As Clarke writes, "The big-four bottled water companies have been highly successful in pitching their message to consumers. Playing on fears of safety and insecurity of water supply, they have been effective in cultivating a consumer culture whereby people become increasingly dependent on buying bottled water to serve their daily hydration needs. In so doing, they have managed to undermine confidence in the public tap water system" (2007, 105).

It was clear to me that no Indonesians had any trust in the tap water. While visiting a zoo, I noticed a girl curiously pushing the button of a drinking fountain, playing with the stream but not daring to take a sip. A sign on the device said "Air minum niagara higienis untuk diminum," which translates to "Niagara fresh water hygienic for drink." Niagara is a private drinking water company whose vision is "to become the best provider of drinking water products in order to protect our customers from polluted and unhealthy drinking water. To deliver high quality products and services to meet customer demands. To support the campaign of conservation and green technology" ("About Us" 2019). I noticed another Niagara drinking fountain on 2 November 2018 while visiting the Gadjah Mada University campus with Endang (figure 9.3). A large sticker on the side indicates "the results of the last test" (*hasil penguian terakhir*) and lists test dates of 1 October and 26 October 2018. Endang said that she rarely saw fellow students using such devices, preferring to fill their personal water bottles from the forty-gallon jugs they feel are more trustworthy.

Niagara is an example of the competition that bottled water companies face from private, for-profit water service companies. The largest of these are Suez, Veolia Environment, and RWE, all headquartered in Europe with North American subsidiaries including United Water, US Filter, and American Water. According to Clarke,

The corporations specialize in taking over public water services from cash strapped governments and running them on a for-profit basis. Contracts often cover a 25–30 year term. In return, these corporations pledge to expand the service and improve the infrastructure. Invariably, water prices are jacked up to cover cost and water meters are installed to control water usage. As a result, millions of people in urban centres have found themselves faced with water cut-offs because they cannot afford the escalating water prices.

The Big-Three water service corporations are getting a helping hand from the bottled water industry in their quest to privatize

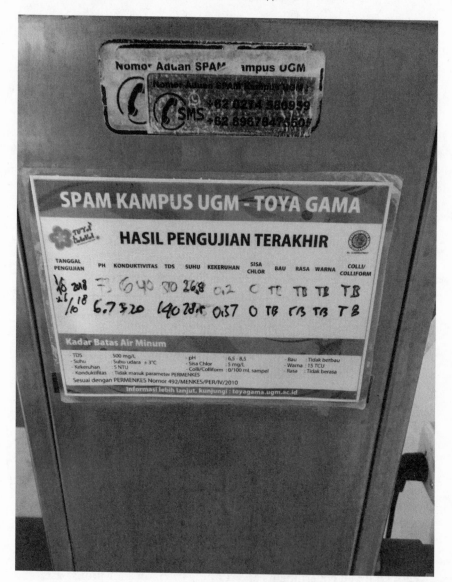

9.3 Water fountain at Gadjah Mada University, Yogyakarta.

water services in North America. After all, the industries' main
competitors continue to be municipal water utilities – and much
of the marketing and advertising for bottled water is designed to
wean people off tap water by undermining their confidence in public
utilities. (2007, 105)

The synergy Clarke describes between private multinational water services, bottled water corporations, national officials, and international aid organizations is perhaps clearer in Indonesia than anywhere else globally. Indonesia was founded as an independent state after throwing off the shackles of Dutch, then Japanese, colonialism. Indonesia's first president, Sukarno, declared independence on 17 August 1945 under what he called a "guided democracy," which promised representative government and social justice for all Indonesians. Article 33 of the Constitution adopted that year states that "the land, the waters and the natural resources within shall be under the powers of the state and shall be used to the greatest benefit of the people." Yet, the promise of public access to clean water has never been realized for the majority of Indonesians. Sukarno's overthrow by the Suharto regime was backed by the United States during the Cold War. Given Indonesia's proximity to Vietnam and China, the United States sought to ensure that Indonesia would not veer towards communism. Like his predecessor, Suharto failed to improve the water supply, but unlike Sukarno he was eager to please Western interests (Vltchek 2012). According to Devina Heriyanto, a journalist for the *Jakarta Post*,

> Jakarta's water was managed by city-owned PT PAM Jaya. However, under the advice of the World Bank, in 1995 then-president Soeharto [Suharto] ordered water privatization, appointing two foreign companies without open bidding. The World Bank believed privatization was the cure for the failure of Jakarta's public water delivery and unequal access to water. Private companies are expected to deliver better management, thus providing the necessary investment for the water company. (2018, n.p.)

Despite the optimism of the World Bank and other neoliberal agencies, private investment has not increased access to clean water in Indonesia. In fact, in 2011 "a lower percentage of people had access to clean water in the major cities of Indonesia than in the cities of India and Bangladesh" (Vltchek 2012, introduction). In 2015, "tap water only covered 60 percent of Jakarta's residents," and yet "tap water only supplies 35 percent of Jakarta's total water demand" (Heriyanto 2018, n.p.). Those without piped water rely on rivers, streams, rainwater, wells, standpipes, bottled water, or other expensive private water sources (Bakker et al. 2006). Even in elite neighbourhoods that had been prioritized in early efforts to pipe in water, many water sources are highly contaminated, as "Jakarta has almost no sewer system; the vast majority of wastewater is disposed directly to rivers, canals, or to (often poorly functioning) septic tanks" (14). As a result, there are high rates of water-related diseases, such as the horrible gastrointestinal illness I experienced on my trip. Diarrhea is the third-highest cause of death in Indonesia and the leading cause of death among infants in the country (Agtini et al. 2005, cited by Bakker et al. 2006).

Given the failure of private companies to meet the targets they had promised, a group of citizens began challenging the constitutionality of privatized water in 2012 on the grounds that it violated Article 33 of the Indonesian Constitution. The case has gone back and forth in the courts, with the citizens winning in 2015, only to have their victory overturned by the Jakarta High Court in 2016 on technicalities. The Supreme Court then ruled in favour of an appeal by the citizens' group for the cessation of private water ownership, ordering "a stop to the privatization of pipe water supply in the city," although the public water company "PAM Jaya has insisted that it would continue to cooperate with the two private companies" (Heriyanto 2018, n.p.).

Although they did not create Indonesia's water crisis, the multinational food corporations that produce bottled water have profited from it. Could there be any better PR campaign for bottled water than when international health authorities, NGOs, feminists, left-wing anti-corporate organizations, right-wing Catholic leaders, and mommy bloggers everywhere denounce formula on the grounds that the tap water is unsafe for babies? Infants require breast milk or formula for around a year, but everyone needs water every day of their lives. The market for water is therefore exponentially larger than the market for infant formula, even if, ounce for ounce, formula is more expensive. It's also the case that there will always be some babies who need formula. Babies must eat, so if the problem with formula is situated in water, then that is even better for the company that sells both the formula and the clean water you need to prepare it with.

I do not have a smoking gun that proves executives at Nestlé or Danone made an explicit deal with the government of Indonesia to mandate breastfeeding in order to drive bottled water sales. It is possible that the rumoured lunch reflected a compromise against the desires of industry, or that the lunch never actually occurred. However, whether these companies supported, opposed, or were indifferent to the law, the reality is that Nestlé's and Danone's water business in Southeast Asia is booming. In

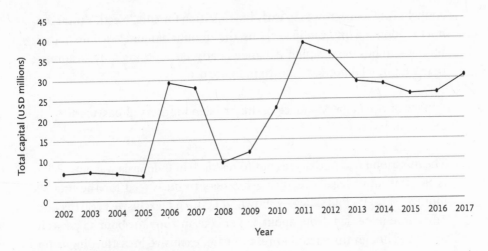

9.4 Nestlé Indonesia capital, 2002–17.

Danone's 2010 annual report, in response to the question "What are your priorities from the global perspective?" CEO Franck Riboud answers,

> We will be sticking to our strategy of focused efforts, investing first and foremost in markets with high growth potential and rapid returns. At Danone, and this may seem an unlikely combination, we call them the MICRUB countries – for Mexico, Indonesia, China, Russia, the US and Brazil. We have been in all these countries for a number of years now, patiently laying a solid foundation that is now rewarding us for our efforts. Our businesses there are posting double-digit growth and they are now big enough to drive the whole group ahead. (Danone 2011, 6)

In Danone's 2014 annual economic and social report, CEO Emmanuel Faber answered the question "Which regions hold the strongest growth potential for Danone?" After noting that Europe was recovering, Faber stated that Africa was "a new frontier for us" and North America was "a key market," and that the company saw "significant growth" in Latin America. He went on to say, "And then there's Asia – led by China and Indonesia – which is definitely a strategic priority for Danone, and where we're continuing to build our water and early life nutrition brands" (Danone 2014, 9). The report notes that Indonesia was second only to China in contributing to Danone's growth in bottled water sales and second to Germany in contributing to its growth in early life nutrition for 2014. Nestlé's total capital in Indonesia (in simplified terms, the amount of money tied up in their Indonesian business) rapidly expanded between 2002 and 2017, according to their annual reports, as shown in figure 9.4.

Impact of the Legal Mandate on Indonesian Mothers' Breastfeeding Experiences

The question I had initially set out to research in Indonesia was this: What is the impact of legally requiring mothers to breastfeed for the first six months of their child's life? As shown in figure 9.5, exclusive breastfeeding rates have increased, from about 32 per cent in 2007 to about 52 per cent in 2017. Though this is an impressive gain, exclusive breastfeeding is nowhere close to universal.

As noted previously, the Qur'an suggests that mothers breastfeed for at least two years, and this is normatively important for most of the largely Muslim population of Indonesian women. According to the AIMI-ASI volunteers, not breastfeeding carries a strong stigma, and mothers who do not breastfeed are seen as abandoning or neglecting their children. Unfortunately, breastfeeding in public is viewed as immodest and is generally taboo, even with a covering. One mother described how uncomfortable many women feel about breastfeeding in public, but quickly noted, "But not me!" as she breastfed her child at the back of the trendy café we were sitting in. I asked, "Did you feel sheepish? Like nervous or shy to do it?" and she answered yes, "at first, but with more practice [pauses] but we have breastfeeding clothes." Someone pointed out that the shirt she was wearing was still open from breastfeeding and we all burst into laughter sharing our own stories of clothing mishaps.

Although Indonesian women may be judged for not breastfeeding, formula carries a kind of cool cachet as a marker of wealth. According to Endang and the AIMI-ASI volunteers, if a mother wanted to give formula, she would be highly unlikely ever to say so explicitly but would instead say that she didn't have enough milk or that there was nipple confusion – providing an excuse for switching to formula without being seen as a bad mother. The volunteers from AIMI-ASI also shared examples of a frustrating lack of progress in getting medical providers to offer more support for breastfeeding. Mothers often reach out to AIMI-ASI seeking help in reestablishing their breastfeeding relationship as a result of nipple confusion

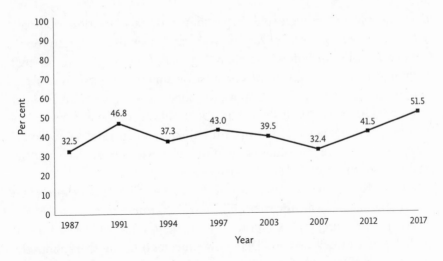

9.5 Percentage of infants aged 0–54 months exclusively breastfed, Indonesia.

caused by giving their babies doctor-recommended bottles. Doctors seem frustratingly unaware or uninterested in helping mothers to breastfeed and continue to receive money or gifts from formula companies. Too often, when breastfeeding isn't working it is formula that is treated as Plan B, rather than referring mothers to a lactation consultant.

The one new mother we interviewed who admitted to never breast-feeding at all shared a heartbreaking example of this problem. This exclusively formula-feeding participant, whom we called Wening, wanted to breastfeed to feel like a good mother. However, she ended up giving birth via a caesarean section in a private hospital near her parents, a few hours from where she lived with her husband. When she came to from the anesthetic, the hospital staff had already started her baby on formula and told her that she could not breastfeed since she had given birth via caesarean, which is a lie. As a result of their actions, she had since suffered from a lot of anxiety and was hesitant to talk to us until a family member promised her that we were nice.

Although Indonesia's breastfeeding mandate has fallen short of some of its aims, one area where it has boosted the success of AIMI-ASI's advocacy has been in informing women of their right to pump their milk at work. This knowledge is only a first step, however, and women still shared stories with us of insufficient space for pumping in many settings. One office removed a lactation room during renovations because it was not seen to be used enough, and we were told that at some hospitals, lactation rooms are available for visitors but not for hospital staff. Given that lactation rooms seemed plentiful in Indonesian shopping malls, this suggests to me that women's lactating bodies are welcome as consumers but less so as workers. An orthopedic veterinarian we spoke to ended up quitting her job in order to breastfeed. She felt that she would not be able to continue to breastfeed and meet the demands of her male-dominated occupation, so she left. I asked if there were any other women in her previous workplace and she said yes, but they were all single without kids.

One of the agency representatives, whom we called Diah, expressed a lot of shame about feeding her child mostly formula rather than exclusively breastfeeding for six months. Her daughter was eight years old at the time of the interview, and Diah now educates other mothers about the importance of breastfeeding. Near the end of our interview, I asked her a hypothetical question:

> Me: Imagine there are two choices – one is that all babies are breast-fed, there's no formula, and the other is that there is clean, fresh water pumped in from the government, which would make people healthier here?
> Diah [no hesitation]: from the breast milk.
> Me [in English to Endang for clarity]: so it's more important that everyone be breastfed, than that … so she's okay with bottled water?
> Diah: [nodding her head]: Yes, ASI.

I asked the same question of the two volunteers from AIMI-ASI-Yogyakarta, whom I am calling Andini and Wulandari. This interview was conducted in two languages; I asked my question in English, and then Endang repeated it in Bahasa Indonesian, to be sure they understood:

> Me: One question I want to ask before I forget, this is a new question from my last interview that I thought of. This is a hypothetical, so just imagining. What do you think would be more helpful for the health of children in Indonesia: if we could somehow wave a magic wand and all babies were breastfed, or alternatively, wave the magic wand and there is clean running tap water for everyone. So, everyone has access to clean running water. What do you think would do more for the health of Indonesians?

[Endang repeats in Bahasa Indonesian]

Andini: For everyone?

Endang: Yeah, water for everyone.

Andini: I think breastfeeding because we distillate water, but breast milk cannot be copied.

Me [to Wulandari]: Do you agree with that?

Wulandari: Of course! [laughs]

They started laughing and talking quickly with Endang and each other in Indonesian. The gist that I captured was that they are used to dealing with the water, but breastfeeding could save lives and the future of Indonesia. This also brought my mind back to a less direct question I had asked in the first interview with a representative of AIMI-ASI. She was making a point about the water being unsafe, so I casually said, why not fix the water? She replied, "That would be too hard."

Fixing the Water Would Be Too Hard

Based on my research, Nestlé and Danone have benefited greatly from the failure of the Indonesian government to address its water problems, and international NGOs have been unwitting accomplices in this. By emphasizing breastfeeding as the "silver bullet" for reducing infant mortality and insisting that formula is unsuitable thanks to the poor water quality, NGOs have been doing free marketing for bottled water. As my interviews revealed, Indonesian women do supplement with formula, whether because of misinformation or disinterest on the part of their doctors or because of struggles such as nipple confusion. And, just like in Canada and the United States, there may also be some women who don't want to breastfeed. All the representatives from AIMI-ASI felt that women *should* have this choice and so their mission is to do everything they can to help women experience success with breastfeeding. Maternity leaves are only three months long, lactation rooms are hard to come by in the workplace, and cultural norms still stigmatize women for being immodest if they breastfeed publicly. In the end, the WHO and Indonesian policies may have convinced women to *say* that they exclusively breastfeed, but the data suggests that they are not actually doing so.

This may also explain why, despite a law mandating breastfeeding, the big multinationals are still tripping over each other to corner the formula market in developing countries. In 2012, Nestlé and Danone were in a major bidding war to buy Pfizer's infant-nutrition business, which Nestlé won by agreeing to pay $11.85 billion. According to a story in the *Wall Street Journal*, this amount is

> as much as 20% more than many analysts had expected the business to fetch. The hard-fought auction shows how Pfizer's nutrition business was seen as a virtual must-have for the two European food giants, which both aspire to lead the fast-growing and economically resilient infant formula business. The Pfizer baby-food unit, while not core to the U.S.-based drug maker, is considered among the world's most attractive given its outsized exposure to developing markets. (Cimilluca, Rockoff, and Das 2012)

Thus, although it has been framed as protecting the health and rights of infants and mothers, the breastfeeding law in Indonesia provides a compelling case study of the use of women's bodies as instruments of the state and capitalist interests. As the responsibility for global health is laid at mothers' breasts, the problem of water access remains unsolved.

10   Taking Moral Failure Seriously

Vann's cell phone rang as he pulled back into the hospital parking lot. It was Kat, Jillian's La Leche League friend. After giving birth to Luna, it seemed like Jillian had distilled her entire identity, siphoned every last drop into a cask labelled mother. Jillian embraced breastfeeding with the fervour of a religious convert, and Kat had slid into Jillian's life as resolutely as the baby had made its way out of Jillian's womb. Vann was mystified by the closeness the two new mothers shared. He would note with a pang of discomfort how much more ebullient his wife's stories were when she relayed them to Kat, how much more embroidered than the scraps Jillian offered up to him. Yet what husband wouldn't want his spouse to be so fulfilled?

Vann recalled one dinner in particular, over too many glasses of wine, when Kat and Jillian had spurred each other's voices to a frenzied pitch. The two husbands had functioned primarily as spectators. The men exchanged understanding nods across the table – their wives were both spitfires, the type of women who came along once in a hundred lifetimes. Glass of wine sloshing as she emphasized each word, Kat had relayed a story about another woman in the League who had made it very clear to her surgeon how important breastfeeding was to her. "So, she wakes up post-op, and guess what. Big fucking shocker – she's been given a completely avoidable medication contraindicated for breast-feeding. By the time the drug clears out of her system a week later, her milk supply has dried up."

Jillian had scowled, then softened her face and reached her hand across the table, nearly knocking over Vann's wine glass. She squeezed his hand. "That would never happen to me with this guy around," she said, winking [referencing the fact that Vann is a doctor]. "Vann's my medical double agent. My holistic fucking superhero." Jillian's face had broken into that reckless smile Vann could never resist, and he had wondered for the millionth time what he had done to deserve the love of a woman like Jillian. And what he might do to lose it.

Vann turned off the engine and brought his cell phone to his ear. Kat bulldozed through a list of questions and concerns about Jillian. Vann answered them as concisely as he could, his eyes on the clock. Visiting hours were almost over.

"Thank Goddess she has you there, Vann," Kat said just before she hung up. "You know better than anyone what's in Jillian's best interests."

Something about Kat's words chafed at Vann as he made his way back into the hospital. "For Jillian," he whispered as he pulled open the hospital door.

Jennifer Farquhar, "Intensive Care"

In the short story "Intensive Care," the Canadian writer, and my dear friend, Jennifer Farquhar fictionalizes the true story of her husband pumping her breast milk while she was in a medically induced coma. Jennifer had barely slept in the seven months since their first child was born and was married to an ER doctor who worked twenty-four-hour shifts at a rural hospital he commuted two hours to get to. She was not only literally exhausted after one of the never-ending hourly feeds she had come to accept as normal but also sick with a virus. Just as her husband was leaving for work, she called out to him for help, her voice barely audible because she was already so ill. The virus she had been fighting turned out to be pneumonia, which turned into a strep infection followed by toxic shock. Most of her organs shut down, and her skin peeled off and her hair fell out once she came back to consciousness eight days later, finding herself unable to walk or speak for weeks. In the fictionalized story, her mother comes to visit her in the hospital one day and starts screaming hysterically after discovering her son-in-law pumping Jillian's breast milk as Jillian lay motionless, only her chest moving with the aid of the ventilator enabling her survival. "You're killing my daughter!" she screams, ripping the breast pump out of his hands. The true story was that the fight involved both of Jennifer's parents and her husband in a big verbal argument at her house while she was on life support in the hospital, though the scene she depicts does make for a bit more of a compelling story for this award-winning novelist.

As Jennifer shared with me, whereas her parents were worried about her being physically depleted by breastfeeding, as a medical doctor her husband

> felt the risk of pumping a few ounces of breastmilk a day was negligible compared to the emotional devastation he thought I would feel once I recovered and learned that I could no longer breastfeed. For him, it wasn't about the benefits to the baby from breastfeeding ... but his concern that I would wake up and be *so shattered* by the fact

that I could no longer breastfeed my seven-month-old baby. (Email to the author, 2 August 2020)

In the end, he did stop pumping her milk and she did eventually come out of the coma and recover fully within a year or so. She has gone on to have two more beautiful children, both of whom she quickly got onto a more formal sleeping schedule, and both of whom were breastfed for a long time. She absolutely loved breastfeeding and did not feel the practice as a moral imperative. As she said to me,

I did believe that breastfeeding was the healthiest choice, both physically and emotionally, for my baby. But there was more to it than that. I really valued the bonding and the relationship that was built over all those hours of having my baby snuggled up against my breasts, her twirling my hair around her pudgy little finger as I stared down at her, watching her feed. I loved the connection that breast-feeding created between my baby and me. And while my colicky baby prevented me from getting much sleep, the breastfeeding part of my caregiving life felt easy and natural to me, and did not cause me pain or stress (complex sleep issues aside), as I know it can for a lot of mothers. (email to the author, 2 August 2020)

This is not simply a titillating anecdote about breastfeeding gone wrong; rather, it strikes me as a symptom of a larger cultural pattern in which breastfeeding becomes disembodied from actual women's lives and needs, raising questions about the lengths to which we are willing to go to see breastfeeding as always best. Though Jennifer frames the situation as the loving act of a husband struggling to know how to support his wife's love of breastfeeding, if we zoom out from the particulars of this family, as a general policy is this what should be recommended? Is breast best when in a coma?

This sounds obscene and absurd; however, we can see actual calls that smack of such a suggestion from the WHO in response to the COVID-19 crisis. I recently read an article on Forbes.com describing research on the ability of the breast milk of women afflicted with COVID-19 to cure the virus (Milling 2020), as though this bodily fluid holds magical medicinal proper-ties waiting to be unlocked by science. In honour of World Breastfeeding Week, the Pan American Health Organization and the WHO produced a

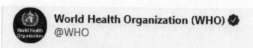 **World Health Organization (WHO)** ✔
@WHO

Replying to @WHO

It is not safer to give infant formula milk to your baby if you have confirmed or suspected #COVID19

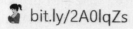 bit.ly/2A0lqZs

#WorldBreastfeedingWeek

If a woman with COVID-19 is too unwell to breastfeed, she can be supported to safely provide her baby with breastmilk in other ways, including by:

Expressing
milk

Enabling women
who have stopped
breastfeeding to
resume
production of
breast milk

Donor
human milk

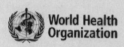 **World Health Organization**

#COVID19 #CORONAVIRUS

👤 WHO EMRO and 9 others

3:46 PM · Aug 1, 2020 · Twitter Web App

10.1 Meme for World Breastfeeding Week, 2020.

meme for moms who get sick with COVID (figure 10.1). No matter how sick or ill mothers are themselves, get out the breast pumps so women can ensure the salvation of others – and be sure never to give formula.

This brings to mind the end of the *Grapes of Wrath*, discussed in chapter 3, in which Rose of Sharon (a.k.a. Rosasharn) nurses the old man in the barn. Apparently oblivious to the reality of breastfeeding, author John Steinbeck imagines this formerly childlike woman reassuringly offering her breast to an old man, telling him "there, there" and then being overcome with a mysterious smile – all of which is ridiculous in real life. Breast milk typically takes days to arrive and, as Rosasharn had given birth mere hours before, she would have only been producing a few drops of sticky colostrum – meaning that the old man would have been suckling at a rather unsatisfying teat. It is unlikely that he would have known what to do with her breast once in his mouth; milk does not simply flow forth from a breast on command and nipples are not some kind of ever-open spigot, spraying buckets of milk. Babies are born with a suckling reflex, but breastfeeding is a learned practice (which is partly why we need lactation consultants). Babies' mouths must be opened wider than one imagines their heads can handle in order to gather enough breast tissue into their mouths to apply pressure on milk ducts that lie inches away from the nipples. Breastfeeding is a mechanical process, not a magical one, and the notion that a starving mother who recently delivered a stillborn child would have the wherewithal to offer healing milk to another adult is both absurd and representative of the myths surrounding breastfeeding.

There was no mention of how hungry Rose of Sharon was or how much hungrier she would be if the book ended just a moment later. As nearly every breastfeeding pamphlet, website, or bit of promotion will tell you, one of the "benefits" of breastfeeding is its ability to deplete calories – five hundred or so per day. The popular breastfeeding and parenting website KellyMom.com suggests that most mothers can lose their baby weight this way and don't need to add any extra food because "when exclusively nursing a young baby, it is very common to feel hungry much of the time ... listen to your body" (Bonyata 2011). How is one supposed to listen to one's body if in a coma, or facing starvation? Breasts will stop producing milk in extreme calorie deficits, after leaching calcium from women's bones and any other nutrients found in the rest of her body. Despite the fables, it wasn't witches stealing milk during the repeated famines of the Middle Ages.

Perhaps recognizing the increased caloric requirements of breast-feeding, the US federal food-aid program Women, Infants, and Children (WIC) changed course in 2009 to offer larger aid packages to mothers who exclusively breastfeed and less formula to mothers who partially breast-feed ("WIC Program" 2018). This change from equal payments to formula-feeding and breastfeeding mothers has been shown to have successfully increased the rate of participants who exclusively breastfeed (Li et al. 2019). However, as political scientist Courtney Jung (2015) points out in her book *Lactivism*, the extra money disappears with any supplementation of formula, even if the mother is still primarily breastfeeding. This policy also subjects mothers to increased state surveillance to ensure that they really are exclusively breastfeeding, which is particularly concerning in a con-text with limited to no maternity leaves and few subsidies for child care. Women may not be able to work and exclusively breastfeed; even if they can, mothers who breastfeed exclusively for six months or more have been shown to experience depressed income in the long term (Rippeyoung and Noonan 2012b).

Even with adequate caloric intake, there remains undeniable evidence that some mothers actually do not produce sufficient milk to feed their babies (Lee and Kelleher 2016). Regardless of how common this problem is, the suggestion that every breastfeeding "failure" can be resolved with more education, better maternity leaves, and more lactation consultants (Singla et al. 2018) puts infants at risk when mothers whose bodies produce too little milk are not believed and lifesaving alternatives are delayed. Further, such suggestions minimize the costs of successful breastfeeding and the power and durability of structural inequalities to limit some mothers' abil-ity to breastfeed. In other words, there are real reasons that many women do not breastfeed, including its costs for both babies and mothers.

Moral Failure

Although there are legitimate reasons why a mother might turn to for-mula, there is little guidance from those in health promotion as to how individuals might deal with "failing" to breastfeed, if these struggles are acknowledged at all. For example, Diane Wiessinger, a lactation consult-ant who co-wrote the eighth edition of La Leche League's handbook, *The Womanly Art of Breastfeeding* (Wiessinger, West, and Pitman 2010), sug-gested in a 1996 editorial titled "Watch Your Language!" that breastfeeding can become the infant feeding norm if we just change how we talk about breastfeeding. After first remarking that "guilt is a concept that many women embrace automatically" (Wiessinger 1996, 2), she recommends that breastfeeding supporters help mothers re-label their feelings of guilt as "regret for opportunities lost" (3). She writes, "We do not feel guilty about having been deprived of a pleasure. The mother who does not breastfeed impairs her own health, increases the difficulty and expense of child rearing, and misses one of life's most delightful relationships. She has lost something basic to her own well-being" (3).

Wiessinger concludes her piece by arguing that all breastfeeding goals are "within the immediate reach of every one of us. All we have to do is ... watch our language" (1996, 4). In other words, the only reason mothers are being denied the inarguable pleasure inherent in breastfeeding is because contemporary rhetoric allows for the normalization of formula feeding through bottles. The only barrier to breastfeeding she acknowledges that cannot be resolved simply by watching our language is malformation in breast tissue, which occurs in only the rarest of cases. By this line of reasoning, insufficient milk resulting from starvation, poverty, stress, trauma, major depression, or coma are not true barriers to breastfeeding; with enough gumption, we can turn the tide on low rates of breastfeeding!

The framing of breastfeeding in moral terms seems tragically unfair, particularly since there are cases in which "failure" is inevitable. Philosopher Lisa Tessman (2010) explores moral failure in general as an essential, but often overlooked, thread when developing normative theories – that is, theories that suggest what one *should* do, rather than simply describing how things are. She suggests that this is a particular problem for feminist, critical race, and other anti-oppression theorists who are interested in developing theories that offer "action-guidance" or direction as to how one can behave to transform the world from a state of injustice to justice. Tessman writes,

> One thing that I want from normative theorizing is for it to enable
> me to witness and comprehend, rather than evade, the failures of
> morality, because I believe there are times when a normative theory
> cannot point triumphantly at anything good or right. I think that
> truly recognizing the fact of oppression entails acknowledging the
> associated failures of morality. I worry that because of the kinds
> of normative theorizing that predominate in the fields of feminist

ethics and social and political theory, moral failure remains hidden behind theorizing that is falsely cheerful about the possibility of moral salvation ...

The insight is that dilemmas are situations where moral wrong-doing or moral failure is unavoidable. Because oppression is a signifi-cant source of dilemmatic moral conditions, and as a result moral failure tends to be ubiquitous under oppression, I want at least some feminist normative theorizing to direct attention to the failures that shape moral life. (798)

Though she is not writing about breastfeeding in particular, Tessman (2010) illuminates a central problem of the moralizing of breastfeeding as "best." Such clichés fail to account for what it means when "breast is im-possible," as their utterers refuse to admit that breast ever *is* impossible. When Wiessinger (1996) cutely suggests that "all we have to do is ... watch our language," she ignores a broad spectrum of oppressive forces that lead to disparate breastfeeding outcomes. Further, by focusing on mindsets and language, Wiessinger seems to believe that telling "unsuccessful" mothers to change how they feel, or at least to stop talking about it, will result in a future cohort of mothers feeling magically happy about breastfeeding. We are not to believe what mothers say, and we should especially ignore bottle-feeding mothers, who, apparently, have been duped, are uninformed, or simply make bad choices. And yet, as Tessman points out, within oppres-sive systems, there can be no good choices, no matter how well informed we are.

Theorizing Morality

According to political theorist and care ethicist Joan Tronto (1993), bound-aries, including those between morality and politics, reason and emo-tion, and public and private life, are not natural but rather are human constructions. Despite such boundaries, morality and politics are not separate and apart in the sense imagined by the democratic concept of separating church from state; they are inherently intertwined. Liberals typically believe that moral reasoning should come first and lead to pol-itical action. Machiavellian types argue that the attainment of power should be one's priority, in order to shape and define morality, and thus politics should come first. In her development of a democratic ethic of care, Tronto makes the case that care can serve as the basis for both morality and politics.

Morality need not be "rational" in a Kantian sense of being detached and autonomous; it can be emotional, drawn from daily life and personal circumstances. We know murder is wrong not simply because we are told so or because we can deduce the logical consequences of a lawless state but also because many of us know viscerally the emotional pain and suffering that comes with the unexpected loss of a loved one. Our capacity to love and care for others shapes our moral compass. Because morality can be drawn from daily life, Tronto further explains, "what will help us to better understand the moral problems that we face is to think about them in concrete terms: who is involved in making decisions, how are they involved, who have they excluded, and who is exercising various forms of privileged irresponsibility" (1993, 170).

My perspective on ethics and moral decision-making is steeped in my discipline, sociology. Émile Durkheim ([1893] 2014), a founding father of sociology, developed the concept of solidarity to explain how societies could function and remain cohesive even during difficult or changing times. Whereas pre-industrial societies were organized around what he called "mechanical solidarity," in which social cohesion emerges from shared experiences such as religion, familial ties, cultural practices, and so on, the rise of industrialism increased the diversity and complexity of communities. To Durkheim, the glue that holds together modern societies is "organic solidarity" – a mutual interdependence among people that forces them to rely on one another for the successful realization of life. We no longer all work a farm to provide for all our needs; through a more specialized division of labour, we depend on the butcher, the baker, and the candlestick maker to get through the daily demands of living. This dependence on others provides us with an interest in behaving morally, because violating social norms threatens our ability to function as a society. Fundamental to Durkheim (and therefore to the sociological perspective) is that the textures of our social structure drive moral reasoning.

What this answers for me, then, is how breastfeeding came to be considered a moral requirement. While some would argue that breastfeeding is inherently moral and society needs change in order to support it, I believe that economic and political practices have shaped our social structure in such a way as to demand breastfeeding as a moral imperative while doing nothing materially to make breastfeeding possible for the majority of mothers. The idea that breast is best – no matter what the evidence says and no matter the cost to the mother – is so deeply entwined within the fabric of our society that we can't even imagine an alternative way to frame the practice than in terms of right and wrong.

Liberalism: Justice, Autonomy, and Neutrality

As explored in previous chapters, contemporary democracies and global organizations like the United Nations and the WHO emerged from the Enlightenment ideals of liberalism. Central to liberalism is the idea that the state (governments) should base its laws on values of equality, autonomy, and neutrality in matters of how one lives one's life, or how one decides what is right (Balint, Eriksson, and Torresi 2018). Classical liberal thinkers like Jean-Jacques Rousseau, John Locke, and John Stuart Mill rejected the divine rights of kings, in which the monarch was argued to be uniquely capable of hearing and carrying out the word of God – and was therefore justified in any manner of exploitation on the basis that it is God's will. For example, during the Middle Ages, through ownership of the land, local lords could extract rents, products, or labour from serfs in addition to taxes and fees in the name of the king, the church, or other members of the ruling elite (Hobson [1894] 1940).

Enlightenment thinkers chipped away at these justifications for increasing the wealth of the nobility and emboldened people to agitate against the increasingly despotic rule of kings. Liberal ideas spawned the American Revolution of 1776 and the French overthrow of Louis XVI and his infamous wife, Marie Antoinette, at the bloody guillotine in 1793. We can see this most famously articulated at the start of the Declaration of Independence, when the founding fathers of the United States established the fundamental values for their emerging nation in 1776; they suggested that the right to be free, unencumbered by the state, in order to pursue what makes one happy is the justification for why a people could abolish one form of government and create a new state. Although the declaration's authors cautioned "prudence" and noted that revolutions should not be fomented over "light and transient causes," they nonetheless insisted that when the violations of such rights and freedoms are great, the people have not only a right but also a duty to overthrow the state. Although these original fathers of the United States saw only White men as capable of the reason required to be responsible for such rights, there is now consensus, at least in principle and in law, that most all adults are entitled to these same rights.

The problem comes when "truths" are less self-evident – when laws must grapple with issues of moral decision-making. The legalization of assisted dying, approval of medical marijuana, and access to abortion are all weighed by democratic legal systems based on a shared moral code in which autonomy and equality are key. For the state to violate these principles, there must be a greater social need that outweighs individuals' rights. For example, those who commit crimes can be imprisoned, and the state can seize private land for public use (with an associated payment to the landowner) on the basis of eminent domain. In the field of public health, freedoms can also be curtailed in "cases of epidemics and similar major threats to public health" (Balint, Eriksson, and Torresi 2018, 310).

We all have learned first-hand the power of the public health apparatus to change social behaviour and perceptions of moral decision-making through the COVID-19 crisis. In deciding to compel individuals to comply with public health guidance, states had to weigh the burdens to those affected with the magnitude of the problem with the goal of "achieving a fair distribution of burdens and respecting autonomy" (Balint, Eriksson, and Torresi 2018, 310). With the exception of Donald Trump in the United States, most heads of state listened to public health warnings and enacted drastic changes to social life. The evidence bore out the experts' advice, and those who treated the restrictions to their autonomy as unjustifiable burdens were more likely to die and/or spread the virus. While public health officials got much of the COVID-19 response right, there were things they got wrong or had to change course on as new evidence emerged.

Regardless of how right they are, as Foucault (1980) discusses, medicine and public health derive their authority from the state and serve as a mechanism of social control. Further, there is an important distinction between public health determinations about epidemics and public health *promotions*, which "typically encourage voluntary changes in behaviour for the benefit of the person's own health (e.g. anti-smoking or antiobesity)," as Balint, Eriksson, and Torresi (2018, 310) point out. They note that breastfeeding straddles epidemiology and promotion, as advocates argue that there is a public health crisis while pushing for voluntary change in mothers' behaviour.

An explicit example of this bridging of "the public good" with encouraging voluntary behaviour can be found in the writing of Michael Latham

(1997), quoted in chapter 1. He contends that a mother's right to breast-feed "should be viewed in terms of ethical, moral or civic interests and duties, not as legal obligations on the mother deriving from legal rights of the infant." Based on this moral foundation, he argues that "states have responsibilities and obligations to respect, protect, support and promote the removal of all obstacles to breastfeeding." The moral responsibility to support mothers to breastfeed is based on his claim that "infants' interests in optimal health and nutrition may be jeopardized if not fed on human breastmilk, or even if not breastfed" (416). Latham is notably careful to frame the jeopardy at play as "optimal health and nutrition" rather than as a question of survival.

Although our survival as mammals depended for millennia on feeding at the breast, most babies today are fed something other than breast milk at some point before they are "supposed" to be. Milk is no longer murder, as was argued in 1939 by early breastfeeding advocate Dr Cicely Williams, since innovations in formula have shifted from canned sweetened con-densed milk to complex formulations developed in modern laboratories. Thus, faced with overall reductions in infant mortality, breastfeeding ad-vocates have needed to find new ways to argue that low breastfeeding rates are a public health crisis – pivoting away from life-or-death claims to a greater focus on "optimal" infant health. As breastfeeding advocate and historian Jacqueline Wolf writes,

In the early twentieth century, when the infant death rate was 13 percent, concerned pediatricians estimated that fifteen artificially fed babies died for every one breastfed baby (Wolf 2001, 1). Since the 1930s, however, after the high infant death rate from diarrhea became insignificant due to the passage of municipal and state laws governing the manufacture and sale of cows' milk, doctors have dismissed low breastfeeding exclusivity and duration rates as incon-sequential. Most physicians came to believe that if formula feeding factored into ill health at all, it contributed only to an increase in trivial childhood illnesses. Recent studies do show that these latter-day doctors were partly right: formula-fed children suffer from significantly more gastrointestinal infections (Mitra and Rabbani 1995; Goldman 2000), respiratory infections (Wright et al. 1995; Scariati, Grummer-Strawn, and Fein 1997), and middle-ear infections (Duncan et al. 1993; Aniansson et al. 1994) than breastfed children. Evidence of increased acute illness among formula-fed children is so strong, in fact, that some researchers argue that the normalization of formula feeding redefined "normal" infant and child health. If children are fully breastfed, these researchers suggest, the "normal" colds, stomachaches, and ear infections of childhood are not inevitable at all. (2006, 400)

Thus, breastfeeding advocacy has shifted from emphasizing survival to emphasizing the elimination of common childhood illnesses. When research pokes holes in scientific claims to the benefits of breastfeeding, purported benefits become harder to measure and increasingly distant from the moment of infant feeding. Studies finding few benefits suggest that the reason for this is because they didn't properly measure exclusive breastfeeding. Without any data to support this, it is common for researchers to assert that it is only when babies are given nary a drop of any other substance for six full months that we can truly see how much of a difference breastfeeding makes for infant outcomes (Jacqueline Wolf 2006). This insistence on perfect adherence positions a mother as putting her child's future at risk when she provides that first sip of artificial human milk, even if her child seems to be doing just fine on formula. In other words, moral failure happens regardless of any negative outcome.

Whether or not breastfeeding optimizes infant health as much as is claimed, for public health breastfeeding promotion to be construed as ethical, the risk to society of not breastfeeding would have to be great enough to override mothers' rights to autonomy and equality. As there is weak evidence that low breastfeeding rates pose the same level of risk as say, the COVID-19 virus, or a measles outbreak, Balint, Eriksson, and Torresi (2018) argue that state-sanctioned breastfeeding promotion violates liberal principles of equality. The language of risk unethically manipulates women into doing something that may actually cause them more harms than benefits, they argue, such as potential risks to mothers' careers, their emotional health, and their ability to break out of oppressive gender roles. Coupled with insufficient evidence that formula feeding represents an actual public health crisis, Balint, Eriksson, and Torresi contend that breastfeeding promotion by the state is an unjustifiable use of state power within a liberal democracy. They go on to suggest three grounds on which liberal theory is violated with breastfeeding promotion:

First, breastfeeding promotion campaigns violate basic tenets of justice. Despite wide disagreement about the exact meaning of justice, there is general agreement that burdens should be distributed fairly and, in particular, in a way that does not create or reinforce gender inequality ... [B]reastfeeding promotion distributes burdens unfairly and creates and reinforces gender inequality. Second, most liberal political theory emphasizes the importance of autonomy, but ... breastfeeding campaigns can undermine or violate autonomy. And third, the promotion of breastfeeding violates state neutrality: the principle that the state should not promote one particular concept of the good, or one particular way of life, over others. (307)

The justification for violating individual women's rights, then, relies on convincing mothers that breastfeeding is best for them and that they really would like it if they were just adequately supported. For example, Latham states, "We can then agree that states have responsibilities and obligations to respect, protect, support and promote the removal of all obstacles to breastfeeding. When this is achieved, it probably will be unusual for infants not to be breastfed" (1997, 416). The North Carolina consortium of feminist breastfeeding advocates follow a similar line of thought when they list the basis of their activism within the following series of "conceptual domains":

The value of breastfeeding and human milk for health
The value of breastfeeding for our global environment
The right to breastfeed
Supporting lactation and access to human milk for all
Advancing support for embodied caregiving and all caregivers
Removing barriers to skilled lactation support
Advancing breastfeeding as a cornerstone of health equity (Smith
    2018, 222)

Each of these breastfeeding promoters seeks to position their cause as relating to freedom and autonomy. The injustice they seek to redress through state-sponsored breastfeeding supports is the denial of access to breastfeeding, the implication being that women would autonomously choose to breastfeed, given its benefits. However, a major problem for their own cause is that if the purported health benefits of breastfeeding and human milk form the foundation of their claims, and if evidence is found that they have actually little impact on health relative to formula, there ceases to be a justification for the other conceptual domains listed.

Resituating Breasts and Breastfeeding from Women's Perspectives

As discussed in the last chapter, rare are claims in breastfeeding debates that women have a right to breastfeed just because they like it, regardless of what it represents or how it serves others' interests (Lane 2014). In making her case that lactivism has tended to justify public breastfeeding as a desexualized practice carried out by the "good mother," Rebecca Lane (2014) draws on feminist theorist Iris Marion Young's work on embodiment. In her book *On Female Body Experience*, Young asks "how women's breasts might be experienced in the absence of an objectifying male gaze" noting that "breasts are a scandal for patriarchy because they disrupt the border between motherhood and sexuality" (2005, n.p.). She begins to answer this question by outlining the ways in which breasts are objectified under a male gaze that fetishizes the breast as a stand-in for the phallus. For instance, she writes, "the 'best' breasts are like the phallus: high, hard, and pointy ... the ideal breasts look like a Barbie's." As a result of male dominance, breasts have come to be defined in terms of their relation to men's or babies' needs, rather than as the territory of women themselves. Young reimagines what breasts could be like if they were reallocated to women: "If we move from the male gaze in which the woman is the Other, the object, solid and definite, to imagine the woman's point of view, the breasted body becomes blurry, mushy, indefinite, multiple, and without clear identity." She goes on to suggest that a female-breasted experience might be deconstructed with the removal of the bra – the device that turns otherwise drooping, sagging, amorphous tissue into the phallic ideal. With release from such confining strictures, freed, braless breasts would experience a more fluid state of movement, as they "sway, jiggle, bounce, ripple," making "a mockery of the ideal 'perfect' breast." Young concludes, "But most scandalous of all, without a bra, the nipples show. Nipples are indecent. Cleavage is good – the more, the better – and we can wear bikinis that barely cover the breasts, but the nipples must be carefully obscured. Even go-go dancers wear pasties. Nipples are no-nos, for they show the breasts to be active and independent zones of sensitivity and eroticism" (n.p.).

I read this call for the subversive power of nipples while in Indonesia and decided to see how it felt not to wear a bra for my twenty-plus-hour travel home. Though in one sense I felt freed and comfortable without the constrictions of straps and hooks and clasps poking and digging into me, I also felt extremely self-conscious. I spent much time thinking about what others were thinking of me as I passed through security on the first leg of the flight from Jakarta to Tokyo. I worried I might be viewed with suspicion, stopped for failing to adequately lock up my weapons of male destruction. Looking back, these feelings seem ridiculous and yet I am unable to shake the sense that living bralessly is too transgressive for me. Images swirled in my mind of what it would feel like emotionally to return to my university classroom without wearing a bra. Unthinkable! And so, I returned to my physically uncomfortable bras, although I enjoyed the opportunity to live life more bralessly while working from home during the COVID-19 quarantine.

Part of what I find so interesting about my short-lived experiment is that I felt less natural and less free with the removal of what could arguably be viewed as the least natural item in my wardrobe. Unlike other articles of clothing that cover, protect, or warm the body, bras are hidden and used to transform the natural shape of the body into an idealized version of itself. I have found bras useful while nursing for providing a device whereby nursing pads can be held in place, keeping my shirt from getting soaked with leaking breast milk, and I can find pleasure in wearing beautiful lacy numbers for a sexual partner, but mostly I find that their value is in helping my breasts stay put, out of sight, out of mind. The notion that I could enjoy my large, bumpy nipples or the drooping, jiggling orbs that are covered in stretchmarks, pin hairs, and a network of bluish veins beneath their white surface feels truly radical.

The time that I most loved and enjoyed my breasts was definitely when I was breastfeeding my third son. They were so full and luscious, and he ate them up hungrily. The joy that came with having an ability to provide him not only with sustenance but with warm, soft pillows against which he could lay his cheek was delicious. In my interviews of lesbian mothers' experiences of breastfeeding, one self-identified butch birthmother shared that breastfeeding gave her a new appreciation for her breasts and even altered her gender identity. She said,

> For me it was just, it gave meaning and purpose to my breasts for the first time and, like, they had a purpose and I finally appreciated them that they were a vehicle for my baby to eat. And we would talk all the time that, like, "Oh my God, this baby has existed this long, wholly because of me and this baby is alive because of what I do" ...
>
> So, we still plan on having more children and I intend to, like, I hope to carry the next baby and so they're [her breasts] just

like, they're in waiting. They're going to have a job again. Um, so I'm hangin' on to them. But, you know … we've talked about if that weren't the case I might consider a reduction. I don't think I would do a removal, but, you know … they're just in the way. And, you know, some butches totally embrace their breasts and I'm just not one of them. But it's been like that my whole life … But with my baby it was … so special (Andrea, first-birth mother, age thirty-two). (Rippey and Falconi 2016, 16)

This mother found breastfeeding undeniably empowering in terms of her body's ability to sustain the life of her child for months. This reminds me of an internet meme that says, "I make milk. What's your superpower?" There is something undeniably powerful to think that the entire human race has existed because of breastfeeding. Other mothers with positive experiences in our study reported that breastfeeding improved their body image and helped them to be "a little more loving towards [themselves] as a person" (Rippey and Falconi 2016, 16). As another mother shared with me, "In a way, it was just sort of a primal, and, like, womanly and embodied in feeding, and I enjoy breastfeeding her and felt really glad that I was able to" (15).

If women's enjoyment and personal desires to breastfeed should matter in considering how to talk about breastfeeding, it is also important to honour and respect the experiences of mothers when negative. As shared in chapter 2, one of the lesbian mothers we interviewed found the experience of breastfeeding her second child excruciating and prayed for someone to tell her to quit. With advice and support from La Leche League, she plodded on for a year since that was what she had done with her firstborn, even though it caused her suffering. The saddest story of breastfeeding failure came from Nicole (pseudonyms were used), the femme-identified partner of butch mom Andrea quoted above. More than a year after Andrea gave birth to their first baby, Nicole gave birth to their second. Despite being a midwife and having a lesbian partner who successfully breastfed for over year, Nicole was unable to establish breastfeeding in full and had to give it up at three and a half months. As we wrote in the paper,

She took supplements, used a supplemental nursing system, to assist the baby to receive adequate nutrition while suckling at the breast, and sought out every possible resource, including help from Jack Newman's internationally recognized breastfeeding clinic in

Toronto, but could not produce sufficient milk for her baby. She
cried softly in the interview when telling her story of when they
decided to switch to formula after three and a half months of trying
to make breastfeeding work. (Rippey and Falconi 2016, 26–7)

Nicole was emotionally devastated by not being able to breastfeed. She
hadn't given up because it was too hard or because she did not have the
right support or the right knowledge; she gave up because otherwise she
would have starved her child.

Given the diversity of meanings of breastfeeding, resituating women's
breasts and breastfeeding in terms of women's experiences is no easy feat.
How are we to agitate for breastfeeding in a way that acknowledges that
the same activity may be empowering for some and horrifying for others?
Is a feminist politics of breastfeeding possible that allows everyone to use
their bodies as they see fit instead of setting up conditions in which "moral
failure" will be inevitable, while dismantling the structures of oppression
that make breastfeeding "success" possible only to the most privileged?
And how can we do so without reducing this politics to simple matters
of choice, shrugging off the reality that barriers to breastfeeding are also
barriers to women's full engagement in public life?

Bernice Hausman (2004) proposes a solution rooted in embodied
maternal practice rather than claims about health imperatives. As Hausman writes,

Breastfeeding is not like a disability or an illness; it is a physiological
relation to another subject who is separate but dependent. Breastfeeding represents a radical, alternative form of embodied subjectivity when compared to the idea of autonomous personhood held up
as ideal in Western societies. Breastfeeding both demonstrates and
enacts an ongoing commitment of the procreative female body to
the well-being of others; it defines a form of ethical relation that is
also a biological relation. This is not to romanticise breastfeeding,
however, as this gift relation is also a form of labour. (276)

I am highly swayed by her arguments that breastfeeding does challenge
traditional power structures and that by forcing open public spaces for
breastfeeding, we force open the public sphere to make space for mothers
and for women in general. However, while breastfeeding as a subject of

inquiry helps us to see the ways in which social life is organized around a disembodied male worker, Hausman argues that advocating for breast-feeding *per se* will help solve the problem – and this aspect of her argument is less persuasive to me. If the way to make inroads into the male world is to be found through breastfeeding, the only way to do this would be to make the case that breastfeeding is important to men for some reason. What history has shown is that men's interest in breastfeeding has been shaped by a desire to control women, and promotion of breastfeeding as a social good does nothing to break this pattern.

Additionally, centralizing breastfeeding within feminist praxis over-emphasizes women as mothers, rather than women as women. Most fundamentally, this sets feminism up to become a politics of failure for all women – the child-free, the breastfeeders, the formula feeders, those without female reproductive organs, and all those in between and beyond. Feminist "choice" theories are equally insufficient to address the injustice of the fact that breastfeeding makes life so difficult for women. In other words, although I believe it is important to be honest about the weak-ness of breastfeeding research, I find it morally insufficient to say "do it or don't, it's up to you" while Black and poor mothers are disproportionately harmed by conditions that make breastfeeding infeasible.

Further, I do not agree that it is helpful to argue that breastfeeding is empowering for women. If this were consistently so, why would so many women have sought alternatives for so long? Wet nurses have been sought by mothers for thousands of years, including among the Babylonians, Egyptians, Greeks, and Romans (Papastavrou et al. 2015). According to Ian Wickes, there is evidence of "feeding vessels from 2000 B.C. onwards [sug-gesting] strongly that animal milk was in fairly common use. Many clay vessels have been found in the graves of Roman infants and some, from the first to the fifth century A.D., have been accurately dated with the aid of coins found along with them" (1953, 155). While these earlier eras were hardly known for being matriarchies, such evidence suggests that women's struggles with breastfeeding are not a modern invention.

Given that both maternalism and liberal choice theories emerged from theories developed by men, an alternative framework is needed to truly liberate women to use their bodies with the same ease that men do. As such, this feminist politics must recognize the value and importance of the nurturing body and relationships, while also taking seriously the ways in which women's labour and bodies have been exploited to their detriment.

For women's bodies and labour to be liberated, breastfeeding should be treated not in moral terms but instead in terms of human need. Access to breastfeeding should be as mundane as the provision of public toilets: an accommodation to human need invisibly pervasive throughout the world. Building on the work of others, 1 argue that a significant leap forward eschews liberalism and maternalism in favour of what 1 call a praxis of humility.

11 A Praxis of Humility

Our family of animals, mammals, is named after us women, yes, the mammary glands. The most remarkable thing about our whole type of animals is our boobs. We know that, men know that and babies definitely know that. In fact, at our first Time's Up meeting I was breast-feeding my daughter at a meeting that not only allowed it but welcomed it and applauded it. But anyway, our boobs are amazing and there is a message in our mammary glands. Many men are behaving like we live in a zero-sum game, that if women get the respect, access, and value they deserve, that men will lose theirs. But we know the lesson of the mammaries: the more milk you give, the more milk you make. The more love you give, the more love you have. And the same can be said of fire: when you light someone else's torch with yours, you don't lose your fire, you just make more light and more heat. So, my last challenge to everyone in this room is to spread your fire. Use your fire to light other women's torches and make more light and more heat for all of us.

Natalie Portman

In October 2018, actress Natalie Portman (2018) spoke those words as a keynote speaker at *Variety* magazine's "Power of Women" event. She was being honoured, at least in part, for her work in the Time's Up movement calling out sexism, including sexual harassment and sexual assault, in Holly-wood and in the wider culture. Portman's speech was a call to arms, recognizing the work of those less famous than her, name-checking some particularly odious offenders in her industry, and inviting all of those listening to fight against gender and racial inequities (Nyren 2018). Portman offers a different, though positive, take on breastfeeding, one not typically employed by those in breastfeeding promotion. Rarely is breastfeeding recognized as "amazing" for its own sake without being attached to instrumentalist goals as to what women with breasts should be doing with them. Portman isn't making a moral or scientific case for whether breast is best, worst, or ho hum. Rather, she draws from her personal perspective as a lactating mother to reveal an incredible capacity of her human body. In so doing, she challenges a typically male view of how the world works, to inspire those around her to support and uplift other women and people of colour at work and in their communities.

By reframing breastfeeding from an instrumental goal to an analogical teaching tool, Portman (2018) also sheds light on a significant problem within most typical conceptualizations of breastfeeding. Whether the focus is on the health benefits of breast milk, a maternalist or social justice right to breastfeeding, or a freedom of choice in feeding, all such arguments are founded on a belief that humans are autonomous individuals and that freedom, defined by one's degree of independence to act, is key to the pursuit of happiness. This privileging of freedom and independence is not unique to breastfeeding promotion, of course; it underlies most contemporary debates in modern democracies. As we saw in the last chapter, we see it propelling the work of the United Nations and the WHO and stated explicitly in the US Declaration of Independence and the US Constitution. Most legislative and judicial systems around the world are based on such ideas. Given its ubiquity, this framing of what is "right" as synonymous with individual freedom can appear so unquestionably true that challenges to its rightness may be chalked up as crazy or even fascist. To question the protection of individuals' inalienable rights is to challenge the notion of human rights. And only fascists and tyrants would disregard human rights.

However, applying the framework of rights to breastfeeding makes little sense considering that infant feeding never involves individuals but rather involves a relationship between two (and often many more) people. A breastfeeder's capacity to produce milk is largely dependent on a baby's (or a machine's) capacity to extract the milk. A mother or chestfeeding father and their infant are more likely to make this work if they have other people, such as another parent, grandparents, or friends, who can support them and care for them as they get their feeding relationship established (McCarter-Spaulding 2008). There are no autonomous individuals when it comes to breastfeeding. Further, if freedom is to be found through one's independence to act, a breastfeeding person can never be free, without abandoning their child or stopping breastfeeding. Thus, if happiness is dependent on freedom, then the breastfeeder is doomed to unhappiness while breastfeeding.

However, although women have long sought alternatives to breast-feeding, suggesting that at least for some women the encumbrances of breastfeeding chafe against an internal desire for freedom, women do it if they must. If they hadn't, none of us would be here. And most importantly, there are also women who have loved breastfeeding and feel empowered by it. This includes my friend Jennifer, who returned from a coma and went on to breastfeed two more children for years, and the founding mother of liberal feminism herself, Mary Wollstonecraft!

If some women truly love breastfeeding and if the vast majority of mothers have been willing to do it, at least until the twentieth century, then logically either breastfeeding transforms mothers into alternative humans who do not need independence to feel happy or independence from others is not actually the key to human happiness. Considering, too, that Jean-Jacques Rousseau was a decidedly unhappy person, as he explored in depth in his autobiographical *Confessions* ([1782] 2004), I'm inclined to go with the latter explanation over the former. There are alternatives to the individual rights approach that are better able to account for the simultaneously powerful, life-sustaining, difficult, emotionally complicated, painful, and mundane act of breastfeeding than the ethically impoverished breast versus bottle wars we find ourselves in today.

Moving beyond Universals

When activist and former slave Sojourner Truth asked a group of White women "Ain't I a woman?" at the Women's Rights Convention in Akron, Ohio, in 1851, she called attention to the inadequacy of the individualizing and universalizing claims of the White feminist movement. Whereas White feminists have long been guilty of making universalizing claims while ignoring the concerns of large groups of women, Black and other antiracist and anticolonial feminists and activists have made the case that patriarchy and misogyny play out in ways that are particular to the target of their oppression. We can see theoretical origins of this in Truth's extemporaneous speech, and these themes are elucidated in the Black feminist Combahee River Collective Statement (1976), discussed in chapter 7. Today, similar ideas are summarized in the concept of "intersectionality," or "intersectional theory," and attributed to the work of Kimberlé Crenshaw (1989). Coming from the field of legal studies, Crenshaw focused on anti-discrimination law to challenge the privileging of White women's experiences within the feminist movement and Black men's experiences within the antiracist movement. She notes that the erasure of Black women from these movements not only marginalizes and harms Black women as people but also "creates a distorted analysis of racism and sexism because the operative conceptions of race and sex become grounded in experiences that actually represent only a subset of a much more complex phenomenon" (140).

Though Crenshaw uses the example of anti-discrimination law, we can see plentiful examples of the failure to consider the intersecting nature of oppression within breastfeeding promotion. For example, those who have simplistically claimed that all women will love breastfeeding if given full supports (e.g., Latham 1997, Wiessinger 1996) have likely not explored the history of breastfeeding in American slavery (Freeman 2018; West and Knight 2017). And, though we have also seen the Aristotelian likening of any woman's breasts as evidence for their closer kinship with animals than men, the consequences of such analogies have not fallen equally across all women's breasts. Some breastfeeding advocates dispute the notion that low rates of breastfeeding in the Black community can be explained by Black women's antipathy towards breastfeeding; rather, they point the finger at a racist healthcare system that has failed to support Black mothers to reach their breastfeeding goals (Allers 2017, Hausman 2003). Thus, we see the creation of the Black Mothers Breastfeeding Association (BMBFA), an organization founded and run by Black women to help Black mothers overcome the barriers to breastfeeding.

It is unnecessary to argue about which factor is most at play for Black women: historical racial trauma or contemporary experiences of racism in health care and society. Just as breastfeeding promotion by itself is unlikely to challenge systemic structures of patriarchy, breastfeeding promotion in Black communities is unlikely to end all forms of White supremacy in general, including police shootings, disproportionate rates of incarceration, inequity in education, employment discrimination, and other forms of institutionalized racism. Thankfully we do not need to choose between dismantling racism and enabling mothers to feed their babies in ways that truly speak to them. We can, and must, do both.

In addition to failing to include many women's specific experiences, rights-based arguments that claim to be rooted in universal experience simply get some things wrong. One example can be found in feminist arguments that housework and caring labour are inherently exploitative (e.g.,

Friedan [1963] 2010). Although allocating responsibility for caring labour to women has undeniably limited women's career progression, care work and the people getting paid to do it (e.g., nannies, maids, sex workers) have been disproportionately stigmatized as dirty and less than fully human because of the devaluing of their work. Given their relative privilege, White Western women have thus been particularly successful among women for rejecting both this work and the stigma associated with it, compared with Black, Indigenous, Latina, Southeast Asian, and other women of colour. Not only is this unfair to the women tasked with these responsibilities, but the assumption that care work is always degrading has also had negative consequences for various communities. For instance, Hazel V. Carby argues that some of the efforts to "liberate" women from "domestic drudgery" (Leghorn and Parker 1981) in developing countries through technological "progress" has failed to free women and in fact led to a disruption in the power derived from women's community networks. Where women once laboured together in the fields, in homes, or in markets, where they had opportunities to share stories and life together, with European intrusion and "advances" they now can stay home, isolated with their machines that do the heavy labour. Carby points out that "it is important not to romanticize the existence of such female support networks, but they do provide a startling contrast to the isolated position of women in the Euro-American nuclear family structure" (2000, 127).

Patricia Hill Collins (2008) has also identified myriad ways in which mothering is a source of power in African American communities. Similarly, when I was in Indonesia, I met a mother who had quit her job in a factory in order to breastfeed her child. She certainly did not express a need to be liberated from the care work she engaged in at home, in order to return to work in a hot factory. While recognizing that women can become vulnerable when their fortunes are tied to a man, it would be a mistake to deny the potential for enjoyment or satisfaction from care work. Such a dismissal of women's experiences degrades care as a practice without doing anything to challenge exploitation within our global care systems. Thus, universalizing theories that see care work as oppressive and freedom from care work as liberation fail to see the historically and geographically particular needs and interests of individual parties.

We can see a similar challenge to universalizing claims within the work of postcolonial theorist Chandra Talpade Mohanty (2003), who has argued that Western feminist efforts to unite women negate significant differences between women rooted in geography, class, ethnicity, race, and other markers of social status. At the same time, she has also cautioned against an overemphasis on difference that would lead us to view the world as composed only of individuals, each with their own unique tale to tell. Rather, like intersectional theorists, Mohanty argues for a recognition of the ways in which various social locations "interact" to create inequitable outcomes. Although individual differences exist among people, where one is socially situated can influence how one experiences the world.

We can see the problem with overemphasizing difference in the seeming consensus that women in "developing" countries should all breastfeed, owing to a lack of clean drinking water. Even feminists who are critical of breastfeeding promotion, such as Joan Wolf (2010), seem to concede that women must be free to choose what to do with their bodies – but this only applies to Western women. Such an attitude offers little critical analysis as to why the water supply is so polluted and inaccessible in so many places around the world, including Indonesia, an archipelago of over seventeen thousand islands with abundant fresh water sources. This approach seems to shrug off women in geographically exploited areas of the world as simply less entitled to the bodily autonomy that women in the West are presumed to have.

In their critiques of the freedom-focused, universalizing rhetoric of liberal feminist theory, Black feminist and postcolonial theorists convey an alternative vision that aligns significantly with a newer body of work known as the "ethics of care." Developed over the past thirty years or so primarily by White women in Canada, the United States, and Europe, care ethics challenges the centrality of individual rights as the guiding metric for ethical decision-making in favour of grounding ethical politics in ensuring that the caring needs of all people are met. Though I have not seen much engagement between the theorists, and care ethicists are more likely to frame their theorizing around defining moral boundaries whereas antiracist and anticolonial theorists are more likely to engage in the pursuit of justice, their ideas are quite similar. Similar to Black feminist and anticolonial feminist theories, care ethicists reject moral universalizing and share a relational ontology in which people are seen as mutually interdependent (Carby 2000; Collins 2008; Mohanty 2003; F. Robinson 2011; Tronto 2009, 2011, 2013).

All three perspectives further emphasize the importance of lived experiences that are situated in particular historical and geographical contexts rather than claiming universality while attending only to the lived experience of the theorist. Black and anticolonial experts are more likely to *actually* do this, whereas much of care ethics is a *theoretical call* to do this. Care ethicists are also attentive to how we can eliminate the degradation of care work by acknowledging human beings' mutual dependence to ensure that we get our caring needs met (Tronto 2013). In so doing, we can reframe care away from being a "woman's" issue and toward being a central part of what defines all human lives. One could suggest that whereas Black feminist and anticolonial theorizing poke holes in classical theorizing by highlighting the ways in which Western theories inadequately capture the human experience, care ethics offers an alternative way of addressing moral questions.

Ethics of Care

The ethics of care perspective first emerged with psychologist Carol Gilligan's (1982) *In a Different Voice*, a critique of Lawrence Kohlberg's dominant psychological theory that all people move through stages of moral development, culminating in a capacity to determine what is "right" based on particular principles of social life. Based on her observations of schoolchildren, Gilligan notes that girls tend to follow a different moral path than boys. Girls tend to be more focused on relations than on principles, with a goal of ensuring that everyone gets their needs met rather than determining one ultimate truth of who or what is right. Although sometimes accused of reifying socially constructed gender differences, Gilligan argues that these are general tendencies, not inherently tied to any particular sex-linked chromosomes, and may be rooted in socialization. More importantly, her observation suggests an alternative theory of justice from that traditionally articulated by male theorists, one that focuses on relations between people and situates moral theorizing in lived experiences rather than detached abstractions.

This theory has been further developed by philosophers and political theorists such as Nel Noddings (1984), Virginia Held (2006), Eva Feder Kittay (2013), Fiona Robinson (2011), and Joan Tronto (1993, 2011, 2013), who see care ethics as a fruitful alternative to liberal notions of individual autonomy, rights, and reason. As political theorist Fiona Robinson clarifies, an ethic of care is comprised of four main characteristics:

> First, it requires a relational ontology ... Second, care ethics involves a focus on attention, responsiveness, and responsibility to the needs of particular others as the substance of morality. Third, it demands a

commitment to addressing moral problems in the historical and spatial contexts of real, lived experiences. Finally, the ethics of care involves a reconceptualization of traditional understandings of the nature of and relationship between the public and private spheres. (2011, 29)

From a feminist ethics of care approach, we can more honestly identify the moralizing claims within breastfeeding promotion and decide whether they make sense within our current culture. When contemporary breastfeeding promotion makes the normative claim that breastfeeding is desirable, preferred, and best, while formula is dangerous or risky, these normative claims become moral claims because of the moral responsibility that parents rightly feel to provide their children with the necessities of life and protect them from harm. Not breastfeeding, therefore, feels wrong – it is experienced as moral failure. No amount of protest among breastfeeding advocates that they are basing their claims in science can take away the impact of "breast is best" rhetoric on those who do not breastfeed.

Instead of evading the moral content of actions by hiding behind a guise of scientific objectivity, feminist ethics of care embraces normative moral questions in order to tease out how we came to a particular moral stance – who benefits from it and who doesn't – in order to better resolve moral problems. Feminist ethics of care shifts political goals from a fight for the protection of individual rights to an assurance of our fundamental needs to care and to be cared for (Noddings 1984). Given the foundational ontological understanding that humans exist in relation to others, and not as individuals, these normative goals are more in keeping with human nature than are claims to individual rights. This perspective offers greater possibilities for meeting the actual needs of infants to be fed while also addressing the concerns of some feminists who take issue with contemporary pressures to breastfeed. Getting there, though, requires a significant shift in thinking, given that rights and freedom-based approaches have served as the foundation of most modern democracies for centuries. However, what has driven these and most other political projects is a more fundamental pursuit that helps explain how we got to our current historical moment.

The Pursuit of Happiness

According to historian Darrin McMahon (2006), the driving question of the great minds of the world has been the pursuit of happiness, beginning with the Greeks quest for *eudaimonia*. Often translated as "the good life," *eudaimonia* is a state of felicity so sublime as to be beyond happiness, free of life's toils. McMahon describes the term as

> indicating a flourishing, favored life ... Comprising the Greek *eu* (good) and *daimon* (god, spirit, demon), eudaimonia thus contains within it a notion of fortune – for to have a good *daimon* on your side, a guiding spirit, is to be lucky – and a notion of divinity, for a *daimon* is an emissary of the gods who watch over each of us, acting invisibly on the Olympians' behalf. (3)

Both McMahon and Hannah Arendt ([1958] 2018) point out that *eudaimonia* is intangible and can only be known at a final reckoning with death. As Arendt writes,

> This unchangeable identity of the person, though disclosing itself intangibly in act and speech, becomes tangible only in the story of the actor's and speaker's life; but as such it can be known, that is, grasped as a palpable entity only after it has come to its end. In other words, human essence – not human nature in general (which does not exist) nor the sum total of qualities and shortcomings in the individual, but the essence of who somebody is – can come into being only when life departs, leaving behind nothing but a story. (2018, chap. 5)

If *eudaimonia* were summarized as happiness, then there can be no living happiness, although the fleeting sensation of happiness may come and go. Thus, the pursuit of happiness/*eudaimonia* is mostly futile, since we won't know if we had it until after we die.

Despite its futility, Arendt ([1958] 2018) views happiness as a "universal *demand*" within our mass culture, a demand tempered by an actual lived "universal *un*happiness." She suggests that the modern demand for happiness is evidence of a labouring society run amok. As she writes, "One of the obvious danger signs that we may be on our way to bringing into existence the idea of the *animal laborans* is the extent to which our whole economy has become a waste economy, in which things must be almost as quickly devoured and discarded as they have appeared in the world, if the process itself is not to come to a sudden catastrophic end" (134). Thus, our modern and futile pursuit of happiness may lead to the downfall of humanity. Lost in modern times is the meaning of action as the means to birth something new, having been replaced by hamster wheels of activity to pass the time.

Not only is the pursuit of happiness futile but, as theorist Sara Ahmed (2010) discusses, it can be used as a tool of oppression. Exploring tropes such as the unhappy housewife, the feminist killjoy, the angry Black woman, and the happy Negro, Ahmed demonstrates how pressure to perform happiness can be used a means to control those who are legitimately pissed off about their circumstances. Black feminist activist Mikki Kendall suggests in her book *Hood Feminism* that anger is an important tool in dismantling White patriarchal supremacy, since "no one has ever freed themselves from oppression by asking nicely" (2020, 369). This is why, as Kendall goes on to write, "demands that the oppressed be calm and polite, that forgiveness come before all else, are fundamentally dehumanizing" (370). To acknowledge the unhappiness of the oppressed would be to undermine an unjust social order. To maintain the status quo, demand that the oppressed pretend to enjoy their lot and vilify those who refuse.

We can see this demand to perform happiness in breastfeeding promotion, along with the denigration of those who fail to validate this framing. When Michael Latham (1997) suggests that every woman would love breastfeeding if given adequate support, he ignores the lengths to which some women go to try to breastfeed only to end up with shredded nipples, jaundiced babies, and a sense of moral failure in the end. Further, through suggestions that breastfeeding will lead not only to healthier babies but to happier mothers, a cleaner environment, and the end of global child poverty, breastfeeding becomes what Ahmed calls a happy object, "as if happiness is what follows proximity to an object" (2010, chap. 1). The whole of future human happiness rests on the breasts of mothers. However, as McMahon points out, the word "happiness" comes from "the Middle English and Old Norse *happ*, meaning chance, fortune, what happens in the world, giving us such words as 'happenstance,' 'haphazard,' 'hapless,' and 'perhaps'" (2006, 11). If we're lucky, breastfeeding might make us happy, but there are no guarantees.

The demand for happiness performances denies voice to the unhappy. As Sara Rushing (2020) points out, "voice is inextricably linked to practices of recognition," which means that having one's voice heard differs based on one's social location, one's class, race, gender, dis/ability, or other statuses embedded in power structures. This is particularly salient within the American healthcare system that she critiques, based on its logic of neoliberalism, as both "individualizing and depersonalizing" (139). In this rationalizing economy, for example, standardized doctor-patient contact time is limited to ten minutes or less, while at the same time the best medical practice is to listen to patients and encourage patient autonomy, leaving patients frustrated, dissatisfied, and angry.

What one does with that frustration, however, is going to differ between people, given that there are also different costs for expressing one's anger, depending on one's social position. The most obvious choices are to speak out or to leave. However, as Rushing summarizes, "The voice option can be costly for the individual actor, in terms of time, money, and energy spent addressing the powers that be with hopes of change ... Exit is less costly, so long as there are sufficient alternative goods and services for the consumer to choose" (2020, 137). To Rushing, and others such as Albert O. Hirschman (1970) and Sara Ahmed (2019), leaving a situation becomes not a form of political *dis*engagement but rather a political act of resistance against that which threatens one's autonomy and humanity.

Thus, within this framework, "failure" to breastfeed may be better framed as "exiting breastfeeding" as a political act of resistance to a legacy of breastfeeding promotion that moralizes motherhood. To be sure, there are undoubtedly some mothers who could use more information on breastfeeding. However, failure to hear the complexity of mothers' voices is unlikely to lead to greater compliance, but rather to increased exit. What Rushing (2020) posits is that despite lip service to patient autonomy, within a neoliberal healthcare system, what is expected in practice is compliance. There is no "choice" for people to make, when only one "right" choice is on offer, especially when the right choice is not available to everyone.

Rushing suggests that a framework more useful than choice for enhancing our agency is a "humility-informed-relational-autonomy" (2020, 4). As she goes on to argue,

> a politically revitalized conception of autonomy must be partnered with humility, not in the sense of quiet complacence in the face of authority, but as recognition of our human and historical limitations insofar as we are given in time, space, and fleshiness ... One particular contribution of my project, then, is to show that humility needs autonomy, a realm of freedom we can identify and pursue despite never being truly independent. Without such autonomy, in the

form of the supported self-direction that feminist philosophers have characterized as relational autonomy, humility would be merely a consolation for relative impotence. And autonomy needs humility, because autonomy is not a one time achievement but an ongoing and fragile process, a project of claiming over and again our lives as our own. Finally, we need both humility and autonomy, as patients and as citizens – two sites of subjectivity that I theorize here as importantly interrelated. (22)

Thus, humility is to Rushing a virtue not simply to facilitate a docile and compliant citizenry but rather as a means to an emancipatory democratic system.

Humility-Informed Relational Autonomy (HIRA)

Humility has traditionally been conceptualized within a limited framework of the Christian tradition, wherein it is a virtue "implicated in not-doing or inaction more than action ... in the form bequeathed by Christian thought and practice, humility appears incompatible with core values of liberal democratic citizenship" (Rushing 2020, 34). Christian humility "entails knowing ourselves to be contemptible, lowly, and capable of anything good only because God has graced us with such achievement" (37). Such a conceptualization of humility has made humility the virtue non grata among the preferred virtues of political philosophers such as Machiavelli, Spinoza, Hume, Mill, and Nietzsche, all of whom saw humility as an impediment to freedom and full civic participation.

Situating his claims on the Christian teachings of Saint Bernard de Clairvaux (curiously the same saint said to have been blessed with Mary's milk squirted onto to his eyes, as depicted in figure 4.2), political scientist Mark Button (2005) rejects this view of humility as anathema to political theorizing. He defines what he calls *democratic* humility as "a cultivated sensitivity toward the incompleteness and contingency of both one's personal moral powers and commitments, and of the particular forms, laws, and institutions that structure one's political and social life with others" (841). In other words, humility need not be associated with humiliation or modesty, but rather with reflexivity, or honest self-appraisal. Rushing (2020) builds on Button's ideas while challenging the notion that humility need be tied to the Christian tradition. As she writes,

While some scholars have concluded that humility is fatally flawed
from the perspective of democratic citizenship-subjectivity, others
argue that it never was, or at least it need not be, associated with
self-abnegation or unquestioning submission to authority. Cleansed
of the connotations of self-denial or blind obedience, they argue,
humility can again become an important virtue; one consistent
with (not at odds with) key components of citizenship. In this vein,
several scholars recently have argued for revitalizing humility as a
self-expansive, generous, and even foundational disposition for contemporary democratic life. This "new humility" is less the opposite
of pride, arrogance, or vanity, and more a corrective against cynicism
and disengagement, on one hand, and domination, on the other. In
this approach, humility is seen as a moral strength, which can emotionally equip us to better engage with our fellow citizens and face
the complexities and uncertainties of collective life with a capacious
and resilient spirit. (2020, 38)

Humility is also implicit, some might say even a key feature, within
the ethics of care in terms of a need to dwell in uncertainty. Gilligan's
(1982) research presented an alternative moral compass to that proposed
by Lawrence Kohlberg, first in his dissertation in 1958 (and, I would say,
eighteenth-century philosophers like Rousseau), who suggested that the
ultimate moral value is one of justice where what is "right" is derived from
abstract objectivity. Whereas Kohlberg (1958, 1981) suggested that girls and
women are morally immature for their reluctance to make absolute judg-
ments of right and wrong, Gilligan showed that they exhibit simply a different moral code, one based on context and relationships. Within care
ethics, humility is thus central in terms of engaging in a moral framework
that situates the self in relation to others and requires attentive listening
to answer moral and political questions.

Rushing develops political humility explicitly by coupling these theories with far older lessons found in the *Analects* by Confucius (2007). As
she writes,

the *Analects* offers numerous lessons on when to exit a corrupt
ruler's court [11.24], how to resist political compromise [9.13], when
to leave a state in protest [15.1], how to properly deliver a deserved
insult [17.20], or when to challenge one who rules by personal whim

[11.17]. In these passages, we can see that humility is the dispositional starting point for undertaking actions in an ethically appropriate way. Humility disposes us to engage with others and our conditions in a way that is neither submissive nor self-righteous. The type of righteous indignation that is grounded in humility, then, can be understood as something of a mean between doing or saying nothing and desiring to be radically transformative and glorious in our deeds. Confucian humility, moreover, not only enables one to properly channel righteous indignation; it *demands* that one express such indignation. The limitations posed by our fate neither absolve us from agency nor justify an exclusive preoccupation with the personal. When we encounter the ways in which we are historically given, finite beings limited in our capacity to simply *will* change, we also recognize the ways in which we are *not* limited, and this calls us ethically to do what we can. (Rushing 2020, 49)

In applying humility to the issue of childbirth practices in the United States, Rushing (2020) makes clear that humility is not simply for individuals or recipients of care but also for providers of care. Within contemporary hospital birth practices, "the humility solicited from [mothers] takes the form of deference to experts and cooperation with the system's logic ... In this version of this conceptual nexus, humility as acquiescence reduces autonomy to picking from a predetermined and limited set of menu items" (80). This is partly why Rushing argues that humility must be coupled with autonomy. Without autonomy, there is nothing liberating or empowering about humbly succumbing to the will of more powerful actors. Rather, all people in relation with each other must be engaged in a "cultivated humility" (80) in which we are genuinely trying to be in a genuine equitable partnership. We take ourselves and our interlocutors off any pedestals and aim to understand rather than expound.

As promising as humility may seem, this virtue does not come easily and is arguably in short supply in our current political realities (Rushing 2020). Conversely, personal autonomy is often fiercely guarded, resulting in anger or exit when threatened, though within the neoliberal healthcare system, true autonomy, too, is less available than we are made to believe. However, even with autonomy, one might wonder why someone would sign up for this particular ethic of humility over other possible ethics. As

Rushing puts it, referencing White (2017), "why would I adopt such an ethos, and what makes that ethos *bear out* in political action?" (2020, 143). Though White (2017) suggests the answer comes from "extremely courageous action," Rushing argues that more important are "indignation and endurance." The battle cry of such a "humility-informed-relational-autonomy" that she explores through her own creation of a figure she acronymically names Hira would be "What the fuck!?" rather than the heroic yawps of the ancients (144). In other words, one finds agency in having the humility to give up on a hopeless but intolerable situation and finds a way to write a new ending to one's story. However, I would suggest that this need for indignation and, especially, endurance suggests that humility may be less of a virtue and more of a "systems-challenging praxis" (Cheyney 2008, cited in Rushing 2020, 136; Singer 1995). Thus, humility is not simply a characteristic of the good but a kind of action.

Praxis and the Human Condition

Though often associated with critical theory or Marxism, praxis in its Aristotelian sense was revived by Hannah Arendt ([1958] 2018) in *The Human Condition*, in which she distinguishes between three primary activities of an active life (*vita activa*): labour, work, and action. Labour involves those activities necessary to reproduce our biological selves (e.g., cooking, cleaning, caring for ourselves); work creates things that ensure a physical record of our lives (e.g., building, making, fabricating); and action refers to the sparks ignited by a privileged few who make history (e.g., inciting, starting, leading). Action, or praxis to Aristotle, was the most esteemed of the three among the Greeks. Labour is most akin to the work of animals and, therefore, could never open humans up to their full potential. Because women birth and breastfeed, Aristotle argued they could never be liberated from their earthly state. This unfortunate reality was why he further suggested that women should be relegated to the mundane caring labours of the world, since they would never be able to transcend them. Men, on the other hand, freed from such drudgery, could transcend their animalistic human natures to create and incite actions to attain the ultimate of the teleological vision: the immortality of a god. Our only means to live on in perpetuity is through the storytelling (*lexis*) of our actions (*praxis*), as Arendt writes:

Men distinguish themselves instead of being merely distinct; they are the modes in which human beings appear to each other, not indeed as physical objects but *qua* men. This appearance, as distinguished from mere bodily existence, rests on initiative, but it is an initiative from which no human being can refrain and still be human. This is true of no other activity in the *vita activa*. Men can live very well without laboring, they can force others to labor for them, and they can very well decide merely to use and enjoy the world of things without themselves adding a single useful object to it; the life of an exploiter or slaveholder and the life of a parasite may be unjust, but they are certainly human. (chap. 5)

This desire to be remembered, or seen as special, or even just seen, is fundamental to the human condition. As Arendt ([1958] 2018) points out, no person is an island. Our sense of self, our identity, our power, is created in and through our relationships with other people. As discussed in chapter 2, this was first discussed by sociologists when Charles Horton Cooley wrote of "the looking-glass self" and was confirmed more recently by neuroscientists in their discovery that mirror neurons in the parietal and frontal lobes of the brain "discharge both when an individual performs a given motor act and when an individual observes someone else performing a similar motor act" (Sinigaglia and Rizzolatti 2011, 64). The implications of this finding radically challenge the assumption that the self and the other are two distinct entities, indicating instead that "our basic sense of self and our basic sense of others [are] both constitutively intertwined with one another" (72). My ability to understand myself and the world around me depends on my relationships with others. This likely explains why we have such a fundamental desire to be remembered as a hero and never a victim or a villain (Saurette and Gordon 2015).

Arendt ([1958] 2018) discusses this quest to attain heroic status as evidenced by the Greek tales of heroism, suggesting that the only requirement for attaining heroic status is to be remembered that way. For example, she argues that Achilles was a hero not because of what he did or who he was, but because someone told his story. She writes,

The hero the story discloses needs no heroic qualities; the word "hero" originally, that is, in Homer, was no more than a name given each free man who participated in the Trojan enterprise and about whom a story could be told. The connotation of courage, which we now feel to be an indispensable quality of the hero, is in fact already present in a willingness to act and speak at all, to insert one's self into the world and begin a story of one's own. And this courage is not necessarily or even primarily related to a willingness to suffer the consequences; courage and even boldness are already present in leaving one's private hiding place and showing who one is, in disclosing and exposing one's self. The extent of this original courage, without which action and speech and therefore, according to the Greeks, freedom, would not be possible at all, is not less great and may even be greater if the "hero" happens to be a coward. (184)

Heroes are thus born not of their individual virtue but by virtue of a relationship – having someone to carry on their story. However, stories do more than just tell us who we are; they also endure, and in so doing, so can we. Arendt explains,

The Greeks' concern with immortality grew out of their experience of an immortal nature and immortal gods which together surrounded the individual lives of mortal men. Imbedded in a cosmos where everything was immortal, mortality was the hallmark of human existence. Men are "the mortals," the only mortal things in existence, because unlike animals they do not exist only as members of a species whose immortal life is guaranteed through procreation. The mortality of men lies in the fact that individual life, with a recognizable life-story from birth to death, rises out of biological life. (18–19)

To transcend death and to transcend nature, then, requires "a recognizable life-story," which is best ensured when there is a concrete trace of one's life – this is partly why such value is placed in art, according to Arendt. Works of art are the objects with the least "use-value" of all manufactured goods but the longest durability. Paintings depicting great men last for hundreds of years, compared with a chair that can only bear the weight of so many seatings.

This is also in part why we humans are more captivated by distinctness than by sameness. Human greatness derives from our actions (our *praxis*), and our actions that appear miraculous or transcendent are those that seem to defy the laws of probability. This is also where Arendt locates a fatal flaw in both historical materialism and positivist interpretations of social life, as they all focus more on larger trends and averages than on exceptions:

> The laws of statistics are valid only where large numbers or long periods are involved, and acts or events can statistically appear only as deviations or fluctuations. The justification of statistics is that deeds and events are rare occurrences in everyday life and in history. Yet the meaningfulness of everyday relationships is disclosed not in everyday life but in rare deeds, just as the significance of a historical period shows itself only in the few events that illuminate it. The application of the law of large numbers and long periods to politics or history signifies nothing less than the wilful obliteration of their very subject matter, and it is a hopeless enterprise to search for meaning in politics or significance in history when everything that is not everyday behavior or automatic trends has been ruled out as immaterial. ([1958] 2018, chap. 2)

Considering that actions that seem to defy the laws of probability are those that appear miraculous or transcendent, only the rare human can achieve such greatness. Gods, of course, are the most obvious party able to do this, but this is why such value is given to *praxis* enacted by mere mortals. *Praxis* sets in motion the unpredictable, improbable, and potentially miraculous. *Praxis* is what leads armies, revolutions, and social transformation. No human can force life on earth to be a certain way, but some humans can light the wick to start explosive change that could lead us towards our teleological pursuit of happiness.

Waiting in the *Vita Activa*

I suggest that breastfeeding points us to a particular framing of women's heroism, while also raising some questions about the notion that the *vita activa* consists of only work, labour, and action. Where would breastfeeding fall within this framework? Though taking time to feed infants can feel laborious and is something necessary for the maintenance of the human species, it can also be extremely pleasurable for the mother and most definitely for the child. One could suggest that this makes breastfeeding an action in the sense of being the start of something new. However, milk comes (or doesn't come) at the end of a months-long chain reaction after a baby is conceived. There are ways to help or hinder the process, but the milk nearly takes on a life of its own once started. Breastfeeding is also not work, at least not as Arendt explains it, because work leads to the fabrication of an object and, importantly, fabrication is always destructive. As she writes,

> Fabrication, the work of *homo faber* [man the worker], consists in reification. Solidity, inherent in all, even the most fragile things, comes from the material worked upon, but this material itself is not simply given and there, like the fruits of field and trees which we may gather or leave alone without changing the household of nature. Material is already a product of human hands which have removed it from its natural location, either killing a life process, as in the case of the tree which must be destroyed in order to provide wood, or interrupting one of nature's slower processes, as in the case of iron, stone, or marble torn out of the womb of earth. This element of violation and violence is present in all fabrication, and *homo faber*, the creator of the human artifice, has always been a destroyer of nature ... The experience of this violence is the most elemental experience of human strength and, therefore, the very opposite of the painful, exhausting effort experienced in sheer labor. (chap. 4)

Breastfeeding springs from nature, not from human strength, though this does not require us to assign moral virtue to the practice. Nature is different from labour or work in that it creates as it consumes. Breathe in oxygen, breathe out carbon dioxide. A tree takes in carbon dioxide and produces oxygen for us to breathe in. As Natalie Portman points out in the epigraph, feed more breast milk, make more breast milk. Work destroys, nature creates.

Further, according to Arendt ([1958] 2018), in factories, workshops, studios, or any other earthbound means of production, even the most creative among us can make only representations of things already in existence. Though we may produce clones of sheep from mammary glands and call them Dolly (Weintraub 2016), such human work products are a facsimile of pre-existing sheep, not the creation of a truly original ruminant. Though artists may seek to create something new, in the words of the Beatles (1967), "there's nothing you can do that can't be done." However, nature does what can't be done by humans. Though all creations share commonalities, every person, tree, or blade of grass is unique.

The one truly original thing that humans can *seem* to create is the birth of new life – an event and a creation startlingly beautiful and always surprising. However, we do not actually create life; rather, we wait for life to be created. Though we might talk about making a baby or going into labour, we actually have very little control over these efforts, and our ownership of our offspring is merely an illusion. We are not creating, but rather waiting, when pregnant or anticipating the arrival of our milk. This is also what we do after planting a seed in the soil or an idea in a student – whenever we teach, mentor, or minister to others. An active life is full of periods of waiting that are not simply about contemplating the meaning of life.

Waiting can also sometimes feel like torture, though such moments are arguably those most important for growth and insight. Archimedes was sitting in a bathtub, not at his desk, when he exclaimed "Eureka!" upon unlocking the law of buoyancy still used by engineers today (D'Angour 2015). Our muscles get stronger not while we're exercising them but in the period after exertion as the body heals the tiny tears we've created in our tissues. The let-down reflex only happens when we relax. Breast milk is less likely to flow when a body is stressed, exhausted, starving, or otherwise struggling, no matter how hard we try. There is action in being forced to wait, an isometric complement to the isotonic exercises of work, labour, and action.

Like action, this kind of waiting always leads to unexpected and unique outcomes, outside of human control. Each new offspring, biological or not, carries a remarkable similarity to its predecessor and yet is an entirely distinct and unique person. Part of what makes babies so fascinating to the human mind is the anticipation of what this new being will look like and who they will "be" when they grow up. In raising children, we experience children becoming themselves in relation to us but not powered by our own will. We are part of their creation, but we are not their creators. This is more than simply labouring for our daily reproductive needs or the fabrication of a useful or beautiful thing; this is also how we can become immortal.

Cult leaders are particularly skilled at this kind of inactive action, deifying themselves through the reflections (and genuflections) of their followers. In scholarly life, professors are judged in part based on who supervised us and where our students end up. We know of Socrates only because his student Plato told his story. The stories were the work of Plato, but Plato was a creation that emerged from Socrates. In short, we engage in this fourth kind of activity when we participate in the developmental process of another being whose destiny is beyond our own control but whose successes or failures may eventually reflect on us.

This effort of waiting for our creations to cook not only brings us immortality but, like action, also has the potential to bring us closer to feeling like a god. And nowhere is this truer than through breastfeeding. Psychologist Melanie Klein's (1946) object relations theory suggests that children's understanding of good and bad begins with the maternal breast. Like religious conceptions of a loving God and a vengeful devil, newborn infants see the good breast as that which nourishes and comforts and the bad breast as a punishing and sadistic force that withholds nourishment. We are revered and feared by our nurslings who see our breasts as all powerful and the centre of their universe. It should be no wonder, then, that men within a patriarchal culture would seek to control the power represented by women's breasts. How else might one be so close to knowing what it is to feel like a god?

This also may explain why breastfeeding can be so fraught for so many mothers. We are not actually gods, no matter what our infants might think. We are mere mortals, and we have limited control over the life into which we bring our children. We do not get to decide if we will like breastfeeding, if we will produce enough milk or too much milk, or whether our babies will sleep through the night or drive us to exhaustion with hourly cries. Though we can read the experts and get support and follow recommendations, none of these actions can ensure a particular outcome. To act without the humility of understanding this is to play a fool by pretending to be a god.

A Praxis of Humility

Whereas labour requires endurance, work requires strength, and action inspiration, this form of activity requires humility; hence, I call it a praxis of humility. This praxis requires accepting that we are neither the creator nor The Creator but rather mere mortals whose immortality will be determined by a final creation over which we have limited control. This is not easy for us ego-driven mortals. Personally, I hate being out of control and letting go of my belief that I oversee my own fate. Humility is thus not simply a virtue but an effort one must practise.

I have noticed humility is a word used on Black Twitter and on the website of the Black Mothers' Breastfeeding Association (BMBFA), but I rarely see White people use this term. White people have gotten very far on this earth without humility, through the destruction of nature to build, conquer, and control. Humility is also an underlying concept found in many Indigenous cultures in North America, in which respect is given to Mother Earth for the bounty she gives. Mi'kmaq Elders Albert and Murdena Marshall have written and spoken extensively, with their friend and collaborator Cheryl Bartlett, about the concept of *etuaptmumk*, or "two-eyed seeing." First developed by Albert Marshall, to bridge the insights of Western science with Indigenous ways of knowing,

> two-eyed seeing grew from the teachings of the late Mi'kmaw spiritual leader, Healer, and chief, Charles Labrador of Acadia First Nation, Nova Scotia, especially with these words: "Go into the forest, you see birch, maple, pine. Look underground and all those trees are holding hands. We as people must do the same." ... Two-eyed seeing is a guiding principle for bringing together different world views, different paradigms. (Marshall, Marshall, and Bartlett 2015, 17)

Whereas Western medicine comes from science, Marshall, Marshall, and Bartlett (2015) explain that Indigenous ways of knowing come from nature.

> Where do understandings that nourish our traditional teachings, our Traditional Knowledges, come from? Mother Earth provides for us, shelters us, feeds us, nourishes us. So, we then must look to her good example for guidance. Our actions toward her must be actions of gratitude. We, too, must be humble, and provide for other living things. We must provide shelter for the vulnerable, medicine for the sick, and nourishment for the hungry. We must always look to Mother Nature to inform us how to live. We do not inform her. (19)

Two-eyed seeing does not suggest that we throw out science but respects the healing gifts of nature from which we can benefit if we take the time to appreciate them. As Marshall, Marshall, and Bartlett write,

In our stories, in our language, it is okay to talk to birds. It is okay to talk to trees. So, you see, it is okay to talk to all beings in our language and sometimes the trees and the birds or others even answer you. If you are downhearted or depressed, go into the forest and listen to the trees. You will hear them whisper, hear the sap running. Just try to interrupt the gentle breezes blowing through the boughs! You can actually make yourself feel better through meditation and intensify your traditional beliefs. (21)

This is not to say that all disease will be cured by a walk in the woods; rather, it acknowledges the limits of the human capacity to control or influence nature. Peace, serenity, and comfort are to be found not when we chop down a tree but when we listen to it. To get the gifts of nature, we must humble ourselves to receive nature's handouts, rather than inflating ourselves to be the more powerful provider.

If we accept that we are powerless over breastfeeding outcomes, we see the futility in moralizing breastfeeding in terms of "success" and "failure." To frame breastfeeding as "success" indicates that trying harder will necessarily yield the desired results. This would place breastfeeding in the domain of work – concerted effort that produces something new while destroying something in the natural world. If breastfeeding is something that women must work for, we must ask ourselves, what parts of nature are we willing to destroy and at what cost?

Parenting books, expert advice, and plain old common sense tell us that we are responsible for our children's welfare. There is truth in this, yet much of what happens is beyond our control; parenting is a unique combination of labour, work, action, and waiting. In a cultural and historical context in which the value of everything we do is determined by productive work or reproductive labour, it should be no wonder that so many parents are coming undone (Watson 2020). Under contemporary capitalism, too many people are deprived of space to rest, to breathe, and to wait for a eureka moment to arrive.

Applying a praxis of humility to breastfeeding does not negate the need for lactation consultants and doctors and nurses to help mothers achieve their breastfeeding goals. However, such supports are necessary to ensure women's relational autonomy, not because breastfeeding is objectively better for babies. We should provide these supports because to do otherwise would be dehumanizing. By the same token, coercing a mother to breastfeed when she finds it offensive to her personhood is also dehumanizing, regardless of how much it might benefit her or her child. A feminist politics of breastfeeding cannot ignore the thousands of years during which men have tried to take possession of women's role in creating life and must reckon with the fact that mothers are not gods manifested in breasted bodies. Mothers are simply not capable of saving the world one breastfed baby at a time, and it would be hubris to ask them to do so.

References

"About Us." 2019. Niagara Water. https://niagara.co.id/about-us.

Agtini, Magdarina D., Rooswanti Soeharno, Murad Lesmana, Narain H. Punjabi, Cyrus Simanjuntak, Ferry Wangsasaputra, Dazwir Nurdin, et al. 2005. "The Burden of Diarrhoea, Shigellosis, and Cholera in North Jakarta, Indonesia: Findings from 24 Months Surveillance." *BMC Infectious Diseases* 5: article 89. https://doi.org/10.1186/1471-2334-5-89.

Ahmed, Sara. 2010. *The Promise of Happiness*. Durham, NC: Duke University Press. Kobo.

– 2019. *What's the Use? On the Uses of Use*. Durham: Duke University Press.

Akre, James. 2010. "Beyond 'Breast Is Best': Next Steps in the Counterrevolution." *Breastfeeding Review: Professional Publication of the Nursing Mothers' Association of Australia* 18, no. 2: 5–9.

Albanesi, Stefania, and Claudia Olivetti. 2016. "Gender Roles and Medical Progress." *Journal of Political Economy* 124, no. 3: 650–95. https://doi.org/10.1086/686035.

Allain, Annelies. 1986. "Introduction: Cicely Williams – A Champion for Breastfeeding." In *Milk and Murder*, by Cicely Williams, n.p. Penang, Malaysia: International Organization of Consumers Unions and International Baby Food Action Network.

Allers, Kimberly Seals. 2017. *The Big Letdown: How Medicine, Big Business, and Feminism Undermine Breastfeeding*. New York: St. Martin's Press.

– 2019. "Dear White Women: Are You behind What's Suppressing Black Breastfeeding Rates?" *Women's eNews*, 26 August 2019. https://womensenews.org/2019/08/dear-white-women-are-you-behind-whats-suppressing-black-breastfeeding-rates.

Aniansson, G., B. Alm, B. Andersson, A. Håkansson, P. Larsson, O. Nylén, H. Peterson, et al. 1994. "A Prospective Cohort Study on Breast-Feeding and Otitis Media in Swedish Infants." *Pediatric Infectious Disease Journal* 13, no. 3: 183–7.

Appiah, Kwame Anthony. 2020. "The Case for Capitalizing the B in Black." *The Atlantic*, 18 June 2020. https://www.theatlantic.com/ideas/archive/2020/06/time-to-capitalize-blackand-white/613159.

Arendt, Hannah. (1958) 2018. *The Human Condition*. 2nd ed. Chicago: University of Chicago Press. Kobo.

Armstrong, Helen C. 1991. "International Recommendations for Consistent Breastfeeding Definitions." *Journal of Human Lactation* 7, no. 2: 51–4. https://doi.org/10.1177/089033449100700201.

Badinter, Elizabeth. 2010. *The Conflict: How Modern Motherhood Undermines the Status of Women.* New York: Metropolitan Books.

Bai, Dorothy Li, Daniel Yee Tak Fong, Kris Yuet Wan Lok, and Marie Tarrant. 2016. "Relationship between the Infant Feeding Preferences of Chinese Mothers' Immediate Social Network and Early Breastfeeding Cessation." *Journal of Human Lactation* 32, 2: 301–8. http://journals.sagepub.com/doi/10.1177/0890334416630537.

Baker, Lindsay Gartman. 2016. "Breastfeeding in the United States: Economic Analyses of Trends and Policies." PhD diss., University of Michigan. ProQuest Dissertations. https://search.proquest.com/docview/1874470044.

Bakker, Karen, Michelle Kooy, Nur Endah Shofiani, and Ernst-Jan Martijn. 2006. "Disconnected: Poverty, Water Supply and Development in Jakarta, Indonesia." Human Development Occasional Papers, HDOCPA-2006-01, Human Development Report Office, United Nations Development Programme. http://hdr.undp.org/sites/default/files/bakker_et_al1.pdf.

Balint, Peter, Lina Eriksson, and Tiziana Torresi. 2018. "State Power and Breastfeeding Promotion: A Critique." *Contemporary Political Theory* 17, no. 3: 306–30. https://doi.org/10.1057/s41296-017-0158-3.

Barston, Suzanne. 2012. *Bottled Up: How the Way We Feed Babies Has Come to Define Motherhood, and Why It Shouldn't.* Berkeley: University of California Press.

Baumslag, Naomi, and Dia L. Michels. 1995. *Milk, Money, and Madness: The Culture and Politics of Breastfeeding.* Westport, CT: Bergin & Garvey.

Bayard, Chantal. 2018. "Les mères célèbres sur Instagram: Ce que nous révèlent leurs mises en scène de l'allaitement." *Enfances, Familles, Générations*, no. 31. https://doi-org.proxy.bib.uottawa.ca/10.7202/1061781ar.

The Beatles. 1967. "All You Need Is Love," by John Lennon and Paul McCartney. 7-inch single. Los Angeles: Capitol Records.

Belfiore, Elizabeth. 1983. "Aristotle's Concept of Praxis in the Poetics." *The Classical Journal* 79, no. 2: 110–24.

Belluck, Pam. 2012. "Hospitals Ditch Formula Samples to Promote Breast-Feeding." *New York Times*, 15 October 2012, Health. https://www.nytimes.com/2012/10/16/health/hospitals-ditch-formula-samples-to-promote-breast-feeding.html.

Ben-Yehuda, Nachman. 1980. "The European Witch Craze of the 14th to 17th Centuries: A Sociologist's Perspective." *American Journal of Sociology* 86, no. 1: 1–31. https://doi.org/10.1086/227200.

Berger, Peter L., and Thomas Luckmann. 1966. *The Social Construction of Reality: A Treatise in the Sociology of Knowledge.* New York: Doubleday.

Betea, Raluca. 2015. "Magical Beliefs for Stealing the Milk of Animals: A Case-Study on the Romanian Villages in Transylvania (18th–19th Centuries)." In *The Ritual Year 10: Magic in Rituals and Rituals in Magic*, edited by Tatiana Minniyakhmetova and Kamila Velkoborská, 444–52. Yearbook of the SIEF (Société Internationale d'Ethnologie et de Folklore) Working Group on the Ritual Year. Innsbruck, Tartu: ELM Scholarly Press. https://www.siefhome.org/downloads/wg/ry/ry10.pdf.

Blum, Linda M. 1999. *At the Breast: Ideologies of Breastfeeding and Motherhood in the Contemporary United States*. Boston: Beacon Press.

Bodek, Evelyn Gordon. 1976. "Salonières and Bluestockings: Educated Obsolescence and Germinating Feminism." *Feminist Studies* 3, no. 3/4: 185–99. https://doi.org/10.2307/3177736.

Bonaccorso, Frank J. 1998. *Bats of Papua New Guinea*. Washington, DC: Conservation International.

Bonyata, Kelly. 2011. "Do Breastfeeding Mothers Need Extra Calories or Fluids?" KellyMom.com, last modified 10 March 2019. https://kellymom.com/nutrition/mothers-diet/mom-calories-fluids.

Botting, Eileen Hunt. 2017. "The Early Rousseau's Egalitarian Feminism: A Philosophical Convergence with Madame Dupin and 'The Critique of the Spirit of the Laws.'" *History of European Ideas* 43, no. 7: 732–44. https://doi.org/10.1080/01916599.2017.1314154.

BPS (Badan Pusat Statistik) [Statistics Indonesia]. 2017. "Average of Net Wage/Salary per Month of Employee by Province and Main Occupation." Last updated 21 December 2017. https://www.bps.go.id/statictable/2016/12/02/1948/rata-rata-upah-gaji-bersih-sebulan-buruh-karyawan-pegawai-menurut-provinsi-dan-jenis-pekerjaan-utama-rupiah-2016.html.

"Breastfeeding: Achieving the New Normal." 2016. Editorial. *The Lancet* 387, no. 10017: 404. https://doi.org/10.1016/S0140-6736(16)00210-5.

Brenner, Athalya. 1999. "The Food of Love: Gendered Food and Food Imagery in the Song of Songs." *Semeia* (March): 101–12.

Briefel, Ronette R., Kathleen Reidy, Vatsala Karwe, and Barbara Devaney. 2004. "Feeding Infants and Toddlers Study: Improvements Needed in Meeting Infant Feeding Recommendations." *Journal of the American Dietetic Association* 104, no. S1: S31–7. https://doi.org/10.1016/j.jada.2003.10.020.

Brinkgreve, Francine. 1997. "Offerings to Durga and Pretiwi in Bali." *Asian Folklore Studies* 56, no. 2: 227–51. https://doi.org/10.2307/1178726.

Brodeur-Doucet, Annie. 2016. "What Is the Impact of Malnutrition on Breastfeeding?" Montreal Diet Dispensary, 1 August 2016. http://www.dispensaire.ca/en/article/impact-of-malnutrition-on-breastfeeding.

Button, Mark. 2005. "'A Monkish Kind of Virtue'? For and against Humility." *Political Theory* 33, no. 6: 840–68. https://doi.org/10.1177/0090591705280525.

BWHBC (Boston Women's Health Book Collective) and Judy Norsigian. 2011. *Our Bodies, Ourselves*. Simon and Schuster.

BWHC (Boston Women's Health Collective). 1970. *Women and Their Bodies.* Booklet.

Campbell, Charlie. 2019. "How a 7-Year-Old Girl Survived Papua New Guinea's Crucible of Sorcery." *Time,* 16 July 2019. https://time.com/longform/papua-new-guinea-witchcraft-justice.

Carby, Hazel V. 2000. "White Woman Listen! Black Feminism and the Boundaries of Sisterhood." In *Black British Culture and Society,* edited by Kwesi Owusu, 82–8. Abingdon, UK: Taylor & Francis. https://doi.org/10.4324/9780203360644_chapter_7.

Carter, Pam. 1995. *Feminism, Breasts, and Breast Feeding.* New York: St. Martin's Press.

CDC (Centers for Disease Control and Prevention). 2020. "Nutrition: Breast-feeding: Recommendations and Benefits." Last modified 8 November 2020. https://www.cdc.gov/nutrition/infantandtoddlernutrition/breastfeeding/recommendations-benefits.html.

CDC/NCHS, National Vital Statistics System. [1969?]. "Death Rates for 60 Selected Causes, by 10-Year Age Groups, Race, and Sex: United States, 1960–67." Table 290. https://www.cdc.gov/nchs/data/dvs/mx196067.pdf.

Challet, Claude-Emmanuelle Centlivres. 2017. "Roman Breastfeeding: Control and Affect." *Arethusa* 50, no. 3: 369–84. https://doi.org/10.1353/are.2017.0013.

Cheyney, Melissa J. 2008. "Homebirth as Systems-Challenging Praxis: Knowledge, Power, and Intimacy in the Birthplace." *Qualitative Health Research* 18, no. 2: 254–67. https://doi.org/10.1177/1049732307312393.

Cimilluca, Dana, Jonathan D. Rockoff, and Anupreeta Das. 2012. "Nestlé Wins Pfizer Auction." *Wall Street Journal.* 24 April 2012. https://www.wsj.com/articles/SB10001424052702303592404577361070078138812.

Clarke, Tony. 2007. *Inside the Bottle: An Exposé of the Bottled Water Industry.* 2nd ed. Ottawa: Canadian Centre for Policy Alternatives.

Cohen, Jonathan. n.d. "Why Milk and Honey." https://www.jonathancohenweb.com/m&h.html.

Collins, Patricia Hill. 2008. *Black Feminist Thought: Knowledge, Consciousness, and the Politics of Empowerment.* 2nd ed. New York: Routledge.

Combahee River Collective. 1976. "Combahee River Collective Statement." http://combaheerivercollective.weebly.com/the-combahee-river-collective-statement.html.

Confucius. 2007. *The Analects of Confucius.* Translated by Burton Watson. Translations from the Asian Classics series. New York: Columbia University Press.

Cooley, Charles Horton. (1902) 2017. *Human Nature and the Social Order.* Social Science Classics Series. London: Routledge. https://doi.org/10.4324/9780203789513.

Cornershop. 1997. "Brimful of Asha," by Tjinder Singh. Track 2 on *When I Was Born for the 7th Time*. London: Wiiija.

Crenshaw, Kimberlé. 1989. "Demarginalizing the Intersection of Race and Sex: A Black Feminist Critique of Antidiscrimination Doctrine, Feminist Theory and Antiracist Politics." *University of Chicago Legal Forum* 1989: 139–68.

Cushing, A.H., J.M. Samet, W.E. Lambert, B.J. Skipper, W.C. Hunt, S.A. Young, and L.C. McLaren. 1998. "Breastfeeding Reduces Risk of Respiratory Illness in Infants." *American Journal of Epidemiology* 147, no. 9: 863–70. https://doi.org/10.1093/oxfordjournals.aje.a009540.

D'Angour, Armand. 2015. "The Real Story behind Archimedes' Eureka!" TED-Ed. YouTube video, 4:41. 13 March 2015. https://www.youtube.com/watch?v=ov86Yki4rf8.

Danone. 2009. *Danone 08: Economic and Social Report*. Paris: Danone. https://www.danone.com/content/dam/danone-corp/danone-com/investors/en-all-publications/2008/integratedreports/AnnualReport_2008.pdf.

– 2011. *Danone 10: Danone Essentials in 2010*. Paris: Danone. https://www.danone.com/content/dam/danone-corp/danone-com/investors/en-all-publications/2010/integratedreports/AnnualReport_2010.pdf.

– 2016. "Danone in Indonesia." Medium. 31 August 2016. https://medium.com/@Danone/danone-in-indonesia-3ce286067eb1.

– 2018. "An Enhanced Portfolio." YouTube video, 0:41. 17 April 2018. https://www.youtube.com/watch?v=pF52l1ktzrl.

DHS (Demographic and Health Surveys). n.d. "STATcompiler." DHS Program, USAID. Accessed 31 July 2020. https://www.statcompiler.com/en.

Derrett, J. Duncan M. 1984. "Whatever Happened to the Land Flowing with Milk and Honey?" *Vigiliae Christianae* 38, no. 2: 178–84. https://doi.org/10.1163/157007284X00178.

Dershowitz, Idan. 2010. "A Land Flowing with Fat and Honey." *Vetus Testamentum* 60, no. 2: 172–6. https://doi.org/10.1163/156853310X486866.

Dettwyler, Katherine A. 1995. "A Time to Wean: The Hominid Blueprint for the Natural Age of Weaning in Modern Human Populations." In *Breastfeeding: Biocultural Perspectives*, edited by Patricia Stuart-Macadam and Katherine A. Dettwyler, 39–74. New York: Aldine de Gruyter.

Devitt, Neal. 1977. "The Transition from Home to Hospital Birth in the United States, 1930–1960." *Birth* 4, no. 2: 47–58. https://doi.org/10.1111/j.1523-536X.1977.tb01207.x.

Dick-Read, Grantly. 1944. *Childbirth without Fear: The Principles and Practice of Natural Childbirth*. New York: Harper.

Dieterich, Christine M., Julia P. Felice, Elizabeth O'Sullivan, and Kathleen M. Rasmussen. 2013. "Breastfeeding and Health Outcomes for the Mother-Infant

Dyad." *Pediatric Clinics of North America* 60, no. 1: 31–48. https://doi.org/10.1016/j.pcl.2012.09.010.

Duca, Lauren. 2016. "Donald Trump Is Gaslighting America." Editorial. *Teen Vogue*, 10 December 2016. https://www.teenvogue.com/story/donald-trump-is-gaslighting-america.

Duncan, Burris, John Ey, Catharine J. Holberg, Anne L. Wright, Fernando D. Martinez, and Lynn M. Taussig. 1993. "Exclusive Breast-Feeding for At Least 4 Months Protects against Otitis Media." *Pediatrics* 91, no. 5: 867–72.

Durkheim, Émile. (1897) 2005. *Suicide: A Study in Sociology*. New York: Routledge.

– (1893) 2014. *The Division of Labor in Society*. New York: Simon and Schuster.

Eckert, Ken. 2009. "Exodus Inverted: A New Look at The Grapes of Wrath." *Religion and the Arts* 13, no. 4: 534–45. https://doi.org/10.1163/156852909X460447.

Emison, Patricia. 1999. "Truth and Bizzarria in an Engraving of Lo Stregozzo." *Art Bulletin* 81, no. 4: 623–36. https://doi.org/10.1080/00043079.1999.10786907.

Ermacora, Davide. 2017. "The Comparative Milk-Suckling Reptile." *Anthropozoologica* 52, no. 1: 59–81. https://doi.org/10.5252/az2017n1a6.

Eslami-Shahrbabaki, Mahin, Delaram Barfeh, and Parvin Eslami-Shahrbabaki. 2015. "Breastfeeding: Neglect or Excessive Support? A Case Report of Child Abuse by a Negligent Heroin-Dependent Mother." *Addiction & Health* 7, nos. 1–2: 92–5.

Etienne, Olivia. 2017. "Tucker Carlson Shuts Down Guest Claiming 'Breastfeeding Is Not Natural' and 'Beautiful.'" *Parent Herald*, 2 May 2017. https://www.parentherald.com/articles/100542/20170502/tucker-carlson-shuts-down-guest-claiming-breastfeeding-natural-beautiful.htm.

Fallon, Victoria May, Joanne Alison Harrold, and Anna Chisholm. 2019. "The Impact of the UK Baby Friendly Initiative on Maternal and Infant Health Outcomes: A Mixed-Methods Systematic Review." *Maternal & Child Nutrition* 15, no. 3:e12778. https://doi.org/10.1111/mcn.12778.

FDA (US Food and Drug Administration). 2018. "FDA Talk Paper: FDA Warns Against Women Using Unapproved Drug, Domperidone, to Increase Milk Production." FDA, November. https://www.fda.gov/drugs/information-drug-class/fda-talk-paper-fda-warns-against-women-using-unapproved-drug-domperidone-increase-milk-production.

Federici, Silvia. 2014. *Caliban and the Witch: Women, the Body and Primitive Accumulation*. 2nd rev. ed. Brooklyn, NY: Autonomedia.

Fein, Sara Beck, and Christina D. Falci. 1999. "Infant Formula Preparation, Handling, and Related Practices in the United States." *Journal of the American Dietetic Association* 99, no. 10: 1234–40. https://doi.org/10.1016/S0002-8223(99)00304-1.

Feltner, Cynthia, Rachel Palmieri Weber, Alison Stuebe, Catherine A. Grodensky, Colin Orr, and Meera Viswanathan. 2018. "Breastfeeding Programs and Policies,

Breastfeeding Uptake, and Maternal Health Outcomes in Developed Countries." Rockville, MD: Agency for Healthcare Research and Quality. http://www.ncbi.nlm.nih.gov/books/NBK525106.

Fewtrell, Mary, Jiri Bronsky, Cristina Campoy, Magnus Domellöf, Nicholas Embleton, Nataša Fidler Mis, Iva Hojsak, et al. 2017. "Complementary Feeding: A Position Paper by the European Society for Paediatric Gastroenterology, Hepatology, and Nutrition (ESPGHAN) Committee on Nutrition." *Journal of Pediatric Gastroenterology and Nutrition* 64, no. 1: 119–32. https://doi.org/10.1097/mpg.0000000000001454.

Fischer, David Hackett. 1996. *The Great Wave: Price Revolutions and the Rhythm of History*. New York: Oxford University Press.

Fornasaro-Donahue, Viviane M., Alison Tovar, Linda Sebelia, and Geoffrey W. Greene. 2014. "Increasing Breastfeeding in WIC Participants: Cost of Formula as a Motivator." *Journal of Nutrition Education and Behavior* 46, no. 6: 560–9. https://doi.org/10.1016/j.jneb.2014.03.003.

Forti, Tova. 2006. "Bee's Honey – from Realia to Metaphor in Biblical Wisdom Literature." *Vetus Testamentum* 56, no. 3: 327–41. https://doi.org/10.1163/156853306778149674.

Foucault, Michel. 1980. *Power/Knowledge: Selected Interviews and Other Writings, 1972–1977*. Edited by Colin Gordon. Translated by Colin Gordon, Leo Marshall, John Mepham, and Kate Soper. New York: Pantheon Books.

Francis, Charles M., Edythe L.P. Anthony, Jennifer A. Brunton, and Thomas H. Kunz. 1994. "Lactation in Male Fruit Bats." *Nature* 367, no. 6465: 691–2. https://doi.org/10.1038/367691a0.

Frank, Lesley. 2020. *Out of Milk: Infant Food Insecurity in a Rich Nation*. Vancouver: UBC Press.

Freeman, Andrea. 2018. "Unmothering Black Women: Formula Feeding as an Incident of Slavery." *Hastings Law Journal* 69, no. 6: 1545–606.

Friedan, Betty. (1963) 2010. *The Feminine Mystique*. New York: W.W. Norton & Company.

Gatrell, Caroline Jane. 2007. "Secrets and Lies: Breastfeeding and Professional Paid Work." *Social Science & Medicine* 65, no. 2: 393–404. https://doi.org/10.1016/j.socscimed.2007.03.017.

Geertz, Clifford. 1973. *The Interpretation of Cultures*. New York: Basic Books.

Gelis, Jacques. 1991. *The History of Childbirth: Fertility, Pregnancy, and Birth in Early Modern Europe*, translated by Rosemary Morris. Cambridge: Polity Press.

Gilligan, Carol. 1982. *In a Different Voice: Psychological Theory and Women's Development*. Cambridge, MA: Harvard University Press.

Goffman, Erving. 1969. *The Presentation of Self in Everyday Life*. London: Allen Lane.

– 1974. *Frame Analysis: An Essay on the Organization of Experience*. Harper Colophon Books. New York: Harper & Row.

Golden, Jonathan M. 2009. *Ancient Canaan and Israel: An Introduction*. New York: Oxford University Press.

Goldin, Claudia. 1988. "Marriage Bars: Discrimination against Married Women Workers, 1920's to 1950's." Working Paper No. 2747, National Bureau of Economic Research, Cambridge, MA, October 1988. https://doi.org/10.3386/w2747.

Goldin, Claudia, and Claudia Olivetti. 2013. "Shocking Labor Supply: A Reassessment of the Role of World War II on Women's Labor Supply." *American Economic Review: Papers & Proceedings* 103, no. 3: 257–62.

Goldman, Armond S. 2000. "Modulation of the Gastrointestinal Tract of Infants by Human Milk: Interfaces and Interactions; An Evolutionary Perspective." *Journal of Nutrition* 130, no. 2: 426S.

Göller, Karl Heinz. 1983. "The Emancipation of Women in Eighteenth-Century English Literature." *Anglia – Zeitschrift Für Englische Philologie* 1983, no. 101: 78–98. https://doi.org/10.1515/angl.1983.1983.101.78.

González-Cossío, Teresa, Jean-Pierre Habicht, Kathleen M. Rasmussen, and Hernán L. Delgado. 1998. "Impact of Food Supplementation during Lactation on Infant Breast-Milk Intake and on the Proportion of Infants Exclusively Breast-Fed." *Journal of Nutrition* 128, no. 10: 1692–702. https://doi.org/10.1093/jn/128.10.1692.

Goodwin, Jeff, James M. Jasper, and Francesca Polletta. 2004. "Emotional Dimensions of Social Movements." In *The Blackwell Companion to Social Movements*, edited by David A. Snow, Sarah A. Soule, Hanspeter Kriesi, and Holly J. McCammon, 413–32. Oxford: Blackwell.

Graham-Harrison, Emma. 2014. "UAE Law Requires Mothers to Breastfeed for First Two Years." *Guardian*, 7 February 2014, World News. http://www.theguardian.com/world/2014/feb/07/uae-law-mothers-breastfeed-first-two-years.

Greiner, Ted. 2000. "The History and Importance of the Innocenti Declaration." Paper presented at Allattamento & Politiche per l'Infanzia: Dieci Anni Dopo La Dichiarazione Degli Innocenti, Istituto degli Innocenti, Florence, 16–17 March 2020.

Hannigan, Tim. 2015. *Brief History of Indonesia: Sultans, Spices, and Tsunamis: The Incredible Story of Southeast Asia's Largest Nation*. Rutland, VT: Tuttle Publishing.

Hausman, Bernice. 2003. *Mother's Milk: Breastfeeding Controversies in American Culture*. New York: Routledge.

– 2004. "The Feminist Politics of Breastfeeding." *Australian Feminist Studies* 19, no. 45: 273–85. https://doi.org/10.1080/0816464042000278963.

Hays, Sharon. 1998. *The Cultural Contradictions of Motherhood*. New Haven, CT: Yale University Press.

Heck, Katherine E., Paula Braveman, Catherine Cubbin, Gilberto F. Chávez, and John L. Kiely. 2006. "Socioeconomic Status and Breastfeeding Initiation among

California Mothers." *Public Health Reports* 121, no. 1: 51–9. https://doi.org/10.1177/003335490612100111.

Held, Virginia. 2006. *The Ethics of Care: Personal, Political, and Global*. Oxford: Oxford University Press.

Heriyanto, Devina. 2018. "What You Need to Know about Jakarta's Water Privatization." *Jakarta Post*, 12 April 2018. https://www.thejakartapost.com/news/2018/04/12/what-you-need-to-know-about-jakartas-water-privatization.html.

Hewlett, Barry S. 1989. "The Cultural Nexus of Aka Father-Infant Bonding." *Natural History* 98, no. 10: 8–16.

Hewlett, Barry S., and Steve Winn. 2014. "Allomaternal Nursing in Humans." *Current Anthropology* 55, no. 2: 200–29. https://doi.org/10.1086/675657.

Hicks, Philip. 2015. "Women Worthies and Feminist Argument in Eighteenth-Century Britain." *Women's History Review* 24, no. 2: 174–90. https://doi.org/10.1080/09612025.2014.945795.

Hirschman, Albert O. 1970. *Exit, Voice, and Loyalty: Responses to Decline in Firms, Organizations, and States*. Cambridge, MA: Harvard University Press. ACLS Humanities Ebook.

Hobson, John A. (1894) 1940. *The Evolution of Modern Capitalism: A Study of Machine Production*. Apple Books. https://books.apple.com/us/book/the-evolution-of-modern-capitalism/id510947039.

Holohan, Meghan. 2014. "Victoria's Secret Store Bans Mom from Breastfeeding." Today, 21 January 2014. https://www.today.com/parents/victorias-secret-store-bans-mom-breastfeeding-2D11968546.

Horsley, Ritta Jo, and Richard A. Horsley. 1987. "On the Trail of the 'Witches': Wise Women, Midwives and the European Witch Hunts." *Women in German Yearbook* 3: 1–28.

Hrdy, Sarah Blaffer. 2009. *Mothers and Others: The Evolutionary Origins of Mutual Understanding*. Cambridge, MA: Belknap Press of Harvard University Press.

Huber, Joan. 2007. *On the Origins of Gender Inequality*. Boulder, CO: Paradigm Publishers.

Hufton, Olwen. 1975. "Women and the Family Economy in Eighteenth-Century France." *French Historical Studies* 9, no. 1: 1–22. https://doi.org/10.2307/286002.

Iavazzo, C.R., C. Trompoukis, I.I. Siempos, and M.E. Falagas. 2009. "The Breast: From Ancient Greek Myths to Hippocrates and Galen." *Reproductive BioMedicine Online* 19 (January): 51–4. https://doi.org/10.1016/S1472-6483(10)60277-5.

Immergut, Matthew, and Peter Kaufman. 2014. "A Sociology of No-Self: Applying Buddhist Social Theory to Symbolic Interaction." *Symbolic Interaction* 37, no. 2: 264–82. https://doi.org/10.1002/symb.90.

Indonesia. 2012. *Government Regulation on the Exclusive Breastfeeding*. Policy No. 33. https://apiycna.org/wp-content/uploads/2014/01/Indonesia_Government-Regulation-no-33-year-2012.pdf.

Indonesia. Ministry of Health. 2013. *Regulation on Infant Formula Milk and Other Baby Products.* Policy No. 39. http://apiycna.org/wp-content/uploads/2014/01/Indonesia_-Decree-of-the-Ministry-of-Health-No-39-Year-2013.pdf.

INFACT (Infant Feeding Action Coalition). 1979. "Nestlé Boycott Endorsements (Partial List)." Senator H. John Heinz III Collection, Legislative Subject Files – 1975–1991, box 361, folder 3, Carnegie Mellon University Archives, Pittsburgh. http://digitalcollections.library.cmu.edu/awweb/awarchive?type=file&item=591612.

INFACT Canada. n.d. "14 Risks of Formula Feeding." Accessed 16 March 2021. http://www.infactcanada.ca/pdf/14-Risks-Small.pdf.

ICCR (Interfaith Center on Corporate Responsibility). Infant Formula Program. 1979. "An INFACT Response to 'The Infant Formula Controversy: A Nestlé View' Distributed by Nestlé at the Governing Board of the National Council of Churches." INFACT. Senator H. John Heinz III Collection, Legislative Subject Files – 1975–1991, box 361, folder 3, Carnegie Mellon University Archives, Pittsburgh.

Jacobs, Andrew. 2018. "Opposition to Breast-Feeding Resolution by U.S. Stuns World Health Officials." *New York Times*, 8 July 2018, Health. https://www.nytimes.com/2018/07/08/health/world-health-breastfeeding-ecuador-trump.html.

Jacobus, Mary. 1992. "Incorruptible Milk: Breast-Feeding and the French Revolution." In *Rebel Daughters: Women and the French Revolution*, edited by Sara E. Melzer and Leslie W. Rabine. New York: Oxford University Press.

Jastrow, Morris, Jr, and George A. Barton. n.d. "Astarte Worship among the Hebrews." JewishEncyclopedia.com. Accessed 21 July 2020. http://www.jewishencyclopedia.com/articles/2048-astarte-worship-among-the-hebrews.

Jelliffe, D.B. 1972. "Commerciogenic Malnutrition?" *Nutrition Reviews* 30, no. 9: 199–205. https://doi.org/10.1111/j.1753-4887.1972.tb04042.x.

Jelliffe, Derrick B., and E.F. Patrice Jelliffe. 1977. "The Infant Food Industry and International Child Health." *International Journal of Health Services* 7, no. 2: 249–54.

Johnson, Douglas A. 1979. "The Nestlé Boycott." INFACT. Senator H. John Heinz III Collection, Legislative Subject Files – 1975–1991, box 361, folder 3, Carnegie Mellon Archives, Pittsburgh.

Jolly, Richard. 2001. "Jim Grant: The Man behind the Vision." In *Jim Grant: UNICEF Visionary*, edited by Peter Adamson, Richard Jolly, and UNICEF, 45–65. Florence: UNICEF Innocenti Research Centre.

Jones, Dorothy. 2001. "Surveying the Promised Land: Elizabeth Jolley's *Milk and Honey*." *Semeia* 88: 97–111.

Jung, Courtney. 2015. *Lactivism: How Feminists and Fundamentalists, Hippies and Yuppies, and Physicians and Politicians Made Breastfeeding Big Business and Bad Policy*. New York: Basic Books.

Kahneman, Daniel. 2011. *Thinking, Fast and Slow*. New York: Farrar, Straus and Giroux.

Kalan, Jonathan. 2014. "Is Pee-Power Really Possible?" BBC Future, 12 March 2014. http://www.bbc.com/future/story/20140312-is-pee-power-really-possible.

Kamen, Henry. 1972. *The Iron Century: Social Change in Europe 1550–1660*. First American Edition. New York: Praeger.

Karraa, Walker. 2012. "Bottled Up: An Interview with Suzie Barston on Her Infant Feeding Experiences and Implications for Birth Professionals." *Connecting the Dots* (blog), Lamaze International. 11 October 2012. https://www.lamaze.org/Connecting-the-Dots/bottled-up-an-interview-with-suzie-barston-on-her-infant-feeding-experiences-and-implications-for-birth-professionals.

Kedrowski, Karen M., and Michael E. Lipscomb. 2008. *Breastfeeding Rights in the United States*. Westport, CT: Praeger.

Keeble, Eilís, and Lucia Kossarova. 2017. *Focus On: Emergency Hospital Care for Children and Young People: What Has Changed in the Past 10 Years?* QualityWatch report. London: Nuffield Trust and Health Foundation.

Kelly, Joan. 1982. "Early Feminist Theory and the 'Querelle Des Femmes,' 1400–1789." *Signs: Journal of Women in Culture and Society* 8, no. 1: 4–28. https://doi.org/10.1086/493940.

Kendall, Mikki. 2020. *Hood Feminism: Notes from the Women White Feminists Forgot*. London: Bloomsbury.

Kerber, Linda. 1976. "The Republican Mother: Women and the Enlightenment – An American Perspective." *American Quarterly* 28, no. 2: 187–205. https://doi.org/10.2307/2712349.

Kissin, Mark W. 1991. "The Patron Saints of Breast Disease." *Australian and New Zealand Journal of Surgery* 61, no. 6: 452–8. https://doi.org/10.1111/j.1445-2197.1991.tb00262.x.

Kittay, Eva Feder. 2013. *Love's Labor: Essays on Women, Equality and Dependency*. New York: Routledge. Ebook.

Klein, Melanie. 1957. *Envy and Gratitude: A Study of Unconscious Sources*. New York: Basic Books.

Kohlberg, Lawrence. 1958. "The Development of Modes of Moral Thinking and Choice in the Years 10 to 16." PhD diss., University of Chicago.

– 1981. *The Philosophy of Moral Development: Moral Stages and the Idea of Justice*. 1st ed. San Francisco: Harper & Row.

Kosman, Admiel. 2004. "The Female Breast and the Male Mouth: A Talmudic Vignette (BT Bava Batra 9a-b)." *Jewish Studies Quarterly* 11, no. 4: 293–312.

Kramer, Heinrich, and James Sprenger. (1486) 1928. *Malleus Maleficarum*. Translated by Montague Summers. Unabridged online reproduction of 1928 edition. http://www.malleusmaleficarum.org/downloads/MalleusAcrobat.pdf.

Krieg, Peter, dir. 1975. *Bottle Babies: A Film*. [Germany]: Teldok Films.

Kuiper, Edith. 2006. "Adam Smith and His Feminist Contemporaries." In *New Voices on Adam Smith*, edited by Leonidas Montes and Eric Schliesser, 62–82. New York: Routledge.

Kukla, Rebecca. 2005. *Mass Hysteria: Medicine, Culture, and Mothers' Bodies*. Explorations in Bioethics and the Medical Humanities. Lanham, MD: Rowman & Littlefield.

– 2006. "Ethics and Ideology in Breastfeeding Advocacy Campaigns." *Hypatia* 21, no. 1: 157–80. https://doi.org/10.1111/j.1527-2001.2006.tb00970.x.

Kunz, Thomas H., and David J. Hosken. 2009. "Male Lactation: Why, Why Not and Is It Care?" *Trends in Ecology & Evolution* 24, no. 2: 80–5. https://doi.org/10.1016/j.tree.2008.09.009.

Kwan, Natalie. 2012. "Woodcuts and Witches: Ulrich Molitor's *De Lamiis et Pythonicis Mulieribus*, 1489–1669." *German History* 30, no. 4: 493–527. https://doi.org/10.1093/gerhis/ghs077.

"La Leche League Canada." n.d. La Leche League Canada. Accessed 13 March 2021. https://www.lllc.ca.

Labbok, Miriam, and Katherine Krasovec. 1990. "Toward Consistency in Breastfeeding Definitions." *Studies in Family Planning* 21, no. 4: 226–30. https://doi.org/10.2307/1966617.

Labbok, Miriam H., Paige Hall Smith, and Emily C. Taylor. 2008. "Breastfeeding and Feminism: A Focus on Reproductive Health, Rights and Justice." *International Breastfeeding Journal* 3, no. 1: 8. https://doi.org/10.1186/1746-4358-3-8.

Ladinsky, Daniel. 2002. *Love Poems from God: Twelve Sacred Voices from the East and West*. New York: Penguin Compass.

Lamberti, Laura M., Christa L. Fischer Walker, Adi Noiman, Cesar Victora, and Robert E. Black. 2011. "Breastfeeding and the Risk for Diarrhea Morbidity and Mortality." *BMC Public Health* 11, no. S3: article S15. https://doi.org/10.1186/1471-2458-11-S3-S15.

Lancaster, Jane B. 1985. "Evolutionary Perspectives on Sex Differences in the Higher Primates." In *Gender and the Life Course*, edited by Alice S. Rossi. New York: Aldine.

Lane, Rebecca. 2014. "Healthy Discretion? Breastfeeding and the Mutual Maintenance of Motherhood and Public Space." *Gender, Place & Culture* 21, no. 2: 195–210. https://doi.org/10.1080/0966369X.2013.791251.

Laslett, Barbara. 1990. "Unfeeling Knowledge: Emotion and Objectivity in the History of Sociology." *Sociological Forum* 5, no. 3: 413–33. https://doi.org/10.1007/bf01115094.

Latham, Michael C. 1997. "Breastfeeding – a Human Rights Issue?" *International Journal of Children's Rights* 5, no. 4: 397–417. https://doi.org/10.1163/15718189720493843.

"Law and Regulations on Breastfeeding." n.d. Better Work Indonesia and AIMI-ASI (Asosiasi Ibu Menyusui Indonesia). https://aimi-asi.org/storage/app/media/pustaka/Better Work Indonesia Breastfeeding Campaigns/BFW Guideline - Law and Regulation.pdf.

Lee, Sooyeon, and Shannon L. Kelleher. 2016. "Biological Underpinnings of Breastfeeding Challenges: The Role of Genetics, Diet, and Environment on Lactation Physiology." *American Journal of Physiology – Endocrinology and Metabolism* 311, no. 2: E405–22. https://doi.org/10.1152/ajpendo.00495.2015.

Leeson, Peter T., and Jacob W. Russ. 2018. "Witch Trials." *Economic Journal* 128, no. 613: 2066–105. https://doi.org/10.1111/ecoj.12498.

Leghorn, Lisa, and Katherine Parker. 1981. *Woman's Worth: Sexual Economics and the World of Women*. Boston: Routledge & Kegan Paul.

Levine, Etan. 2000. "The Land of Milk and Honey." *Journal for the Study of the Old Testament* 25, no. 87: 43–57. https://doi.org/10.1177/030908920002508703.

Levy, Lauren. 2017. "Mom Films Epic PSA after Being Shamed for Breastfeeding at Victoria's Secret." *CafeMom* (blog). 27 November 2017. https://thestir.cafemom.com/parenting_news/208954/mom-breastfeeding-victorias-secret.

Li, Kelin, Ming Wen, Megan Reynolds, and Qi Zhang. 2019. "WIC Participation and Breastfeeding after the 2009 WIC Revision: A Propensity Score Approach." *International Journal of Environmental Research and Public Health* 16, no. 15: article 2645. https://doi.org/10.3390/ijerph16152645.

Locke, John. 1690. *Two Treatises of Government: in the Former, the False Principles, and Foundation of Sir Robert Filmer, and His Followers, Are Detected and Overthrown. The Latter Is an Essay Concerning the True Original, Extent, and the End of Civil Government*. London: A. Churchill.

Maisels, M. Jeffrey. 2010. "Screening and Early Postnatal Management Strategies to Prevent Hazardous Hyperbilirubinemia in Newborns of 35 or More Weeks of Gestation." *Seminars in Fetal and Neonatal Medicine* 15, no. 3: 129–35. https://doi.org/10.1016/j.siny.2009.10.004.

– 2015. "Managing the Jaundiced Newborn: A Persistent Challenge." *CMAJ* 187, no. 5: 335–43. https://doi.org/10.1503/cmaj.122117.

Marshall, Murdena, Albert Marshall, and Cheryl Bartlett. 2015. "Two-Eyed Seeing in Medicine." In *Determinants of Indigenous Peoples' Health*, edited by Margo Greenwood, Sarah De Leeuw, Nicole Marie Lindsay, and Charlotte Reading. Toronto: Canadian Scholars' Press.

Martin, Joyce A., Brady E. Hamilton, Michelle J.K. Osterman, and Anne K. Driscoll. 2019. "Births: Final Data for 2018." *National Vital Statistics Reports* 68, no. 13: 47.

Martucci, Jessica, and Anne Barnhill. 2016. "Unintended Consequences of Invoking the 'Natural' in Breastfeeding Promotion." *Pediatrics* 137, no. 4:e20154154. https://doi.org/10.1542/peds.2015-4154.

Marx, Karl. (1867) 1977. *Capital: A Critique of Political Economy*. New York: Vintage Books.

Mason, Frances, Kathryn Rawe, and Simon Wright. 2013. *Superfood for Babies: How Overcoming Barriers to Breastfeeding Will Save Children's Lives*. London: Save the Children. http://www.savethechildren.org.uk/resources/online-library/superfood-babies.

McCarter-Spaulding, Deborah. 2008. "Is Breastfeeding Fair? Tensions in Feminist Perspectives on Breastfeeding and the Family." *Journal of Human Lactation* 24, no. 2: 206–12. https://doi.org/10.1177/0890334408316076.

McMahon, Darrin M. 2006. *Happiness: A History*. New York: Atlantic Monthly Press.

McNiel, Melinda E., Miriam H. Labbok, and Sheryl W. Abrahams. 2010. "What Are the Risks Associated with Formula Feeding? A Re-analysis and Review." *Breastfeeding Review: Professional Publication of the Nursing Mothers' Association of Australia* 18, no. 2: 25–32.

Mead, George Herbert. (1934) 2015. *Mind, Self, and Society: The Definitive Edition*. Edited by Charles W. Morris. Chicago: University of Chicago Press.

Michelson, Marcel and Reed Stevenson. 2007. "Danone Offers $17 Bln for Food Firm Numico." *Reuters*, 9 July 2007. https://www.reuters.com/article/us-danone-numico-idusweb467920070709.

Milling, Marla. 2020. "Breast Milk Studied as Potential Coronavirus Treatment." *Forbes*, 24 April 2020, Innovation. https://www.forbes.com/sites/marlamilling/2020/04/24/breast-milk-studied-as-potential-coronavirus-treatment.

Mitra, Amal K., and Fauziah Rabbani. 1995. "The Importance of Breastfeeding in Minimizing Mortality and Morbidity from Diarrhoeal Diseases: The Bangladesh Perspective." *Journal of Diarrhoeal Diseases Research* 13, no. 1: 1–7.

Mohanty, Chandra Talpade. 2003. "'Under Western Eyes' Revisited: Feminist Solidarity through Anticapitalist Struggles." *Signs: Journal of Women in Culture and Society* 28, no. 2: 499–535.

Muller, Mike. 1974. "The Baby Killer." London: War on Want. https://waronwant.org/sites/default/files/THE%20BABY%20KILLER%201974.pdf.

Murphy, Rita Catherine. 2012. "The Facts of Infact: How the Infant Formula Controversy Went from a Public Health Crisis to an International Consumer Activist Issue." Master's thesis, University of Minnesota. https://conservancy.umn.edu/bitstream/handle/11299/130941/1/Murphy_Rita_May2012.pdf.

Nathoo, Tasnim, and Aleck Ostry. 2009. *The One Best Way? Breastfeeding History, Politics, and Policy in Canada*. Waterloo, ON: Wilfrid Laurier University Press.

Neifert, Marianne R. 2001. "Prevention of Breastfeeding Tragedies." *Pediatric Clinics* 48, no. 2: 273–97. https://doi.org/10.1016/s0031-3955(08)70026-9.

Nelson, Jennifer M., and Daurice A. Grossniklaus. 2019. "Trends in Hospital Breastfeeding Policies in the United States from 2009–2015: Results from the Maternity Practices in Infant Nutrition and Care Survey." *Breastfeeding Medicine* 14, no. 3: 165–71. https://doi.org/10.1089/bfm.2018.0224.

Nestlé. 2008. "2007 Financial Statements: Consolidated Financial Statements of the Nestlé Group." https://www.nestle.com/asset-library/documents/library/documents/financial_statements/2007-financial-statements-en.pdf.

"The Nestlé Company History." n.d. Nestlé Global. Accessed 8 March 2021. https://www.nestle.com/aboutus/history/nestle-company-history.

NIDDK (National Institute of Diabetes and Digestive and Kidney Diseases). 2017. "Overweight & Obesity Statistics." August 2017. https://www.niddk.nih.gov/health-information/health-statistics/overweight-obesity.

Nik-Khah, Edward, and Robert Van Horn. 2016. "The Ascendancy of Chicago Neoliberalism." In *The Handbook of Neoliberalism*, edited by Simon Springer, Kean Birch, and Julie MacLeavy, 27–38. New York: Routledge.

Noddings, Nel. 1984. *Caring: A Feminine Approach to Ethics and Moral Education*. Berkeley: University of California Press.

Norris, Jill M., Katherine Barriga, Georgeanna Klingensmith, Michelle Hoffman, George S. Eisenbarth, Henry A. Erlich, and Marian Rewers. 2003. "Timing of Initial Cereal Exposure in Infancy and Risk of Islet Autoimmunity." *JAMA* 290, no. 13: 1713–20. https://doi.org/10.1001/jama.290.13.1713.

Nyi Nyi. 2001. "Building Foundations for Castles in the Air." In *Jim Grant: UNICEF Visionary*, edited by Peter Adamson, Richard Jolly, and UNICEF, 67–86. Florence: UNICEF Innocenti Research Centre.

Nyren, Erin. 2018. "Natalie Portman's Step-by-Step Guide on How to Topple the Patriarchy (Watch)." Variety.com. 12 October. https://variety.com/2018/film/news/natalie-portman-gender-parity-power-of-women-1202978582.

O'Connor, Nina R., Kawai O. Tanabe, Mir S. Siadaty, and Fern R. Hauck. 2009. "Pacifiers and Breastfeeding: A Systematic Review." *Archives of Pediatrics & Adolescent Medicine* 163, no. 4: 378–82. https://doi.org/10.1001/archpediatrics.2008.578.

"Our Epic History." n.d. Danone. Accessed 17 March 2021. https://www.danone.com/about-danone/ourhistory.html.

"Our Mission." 2018. International Baby Food Action Network (IBFAN). Accessed 17 March 2021. https://www.ibfan.org/our-mission-2.

"Our Story." n.d. Our Bodies Ourselves. Accessed 15 March 2021. https://www.ourbodiesourselves.org/our-story.

Packer, Craig, Susan Lewis, and Anne Pusey. 1992. "A Comparative Analysis of Non-Offspring Nursing." *Animal Behaviour* 43, no. 2: 265–81. https://doi.org/10.1016/S0003-3472(05)80222-2.

PAHO/WHO (Pan American Health Organization/World Health Organization). 2016. "New Evidence in The Lancet Shows More Benefits of Breastfeeding." Press release. 30 January 2016. https://www.paho.org/hq/index.php?option= com_content&view=article&id=11634:2016-new-evidence-in-shows-more-benefits-breastfeeding&Itemid=1926&lang=en.

Papastavrou, M., S.M. Genitsaridi, E. Komodiki, S. Paliatsou, A. Kontogeorgou, and Nicoletta Iacovidou. 2015. "Breastfeeding in the Course of History." *Journal of Pediatrics & Neonatal Care* 2, no. 6: 00096. https://doi.org/10.15406/jpnc.2015. 02.00096.

Parinetto, Luciano. 1998. *Streghe e potere: Il capitale e la persecuzione dei diversi.* Milan: Rusconi.

Pisacane, Alfredo, Paola Continisio, Orsola Palma, Stefania Cataldo, Fabiola De Michele, and Ugo Vairo. 2010. "Breastfeeding and Risk for Fever after Immunization." *Pediatrics* 125, no. 6: e1448–52. https://doi.org/10.1542/peds.2009-1911.

Pope, Carley J., and Dwight Mazmanian. 2016. "Breastfeeding and Postpartum Depression: An Overview and Methodological Recommendations for Future Research." *Depression Research and Treatment* 2016: article 4765310. https://doi.org/ 10.1155/2016/4765310.

Popper, Karl. (1959) 2005. *The Logic of Scientific Discovery.* London: Routledge. Ebook.

Portman, Natalie. 2018. "Natalie Portman's Step-by-Step Guide to Toppling the Patriarchy." Speech at Variety Power of Women Event, Los Angeles. YouTube video, 15:35. 12 October. https://www.youtube.com/watch?v=oqukNm3Bhgg.

Public Health Agency of Canada. 2021. "Breastfeeding." In *Family-Centred Maternity and Newborn Care: National Guidelines*, chap. 6. Last modified 4 February 2021. https://www.canada.ca/en/public-health/services/publications/healthy-living/maternity-newborn-care-guidelines-chapter-6.html.

Quigley, Maria A., Yvonne J. Kelly, and Amanda Sacker. 2007. "Breastfeeding and Hospitalization for Diarrheal and Respiratory Infection in the United Kingdom Millennium Cohort Study." *Pediatrics* 119, no. 4: e837–42. https://doi.org/ 10.1542/peds.2006-2256.

Racelis, Mary. 2001. "Controversy and Continuity: Programming for Women in Jim Grant's UNICEF." In *Jim Grant: UNICEF Visionary*, edited by Peter Adamson, Richard Jolly, and UNICEF, 111–35. Florence: UNICEF Innocenti Research Centre.

Racey, Daniel N., Malcolm Peaker, and Paul A. Racey. 2009. "Galactorrhoea Is Not Lactation." *Trends in Ecology & Evolution* 24, no. 7: 354–5; author reply 355. https://doi.org/10.1016/j.tree.2009.03.008.

Remembering Mother Florence Leung. 2017. "2 months have passed since the Detectives and victim assistance staffs showed up at our home." Facebook, 17 January 2017. https://www.facebook.com/prayforflo/posts/1839681439653483.

Richards, Cynthia. 2009. "The Body of Her Work, the Work of Her Body: Accounting for the Life and Death of Mary Wollstonecraft." *Eighteenth-Century Fiction* 21, no. 4: 565–92. https://doi.org/10.3138/ecf.21.4.565.

Rippey, Phyllis L.F., Fabiola Aravena, and John Paul Nyonator. 2020. "Health Impacts of Early Complementary Food Introduction between Formula-Fed and Breastfed Infants." *Journal of Pediatric Gastroenterology and Nutrition* 70, no. 3: 375–80.

Rippey, Phyllis L.F., and Laurel Falconi. 2016. "A Land of Milk and Honey? Breastfeeding and Identity in Lesbian Families." *Journal of GLBT Family Studies* 13, no. 1: 16–39. https://doi.org/10.1080/1550428X.2015.1129297.

Rippeyoung, Phyllis L.F., and Mary C. Noonan. 2012a. "Breastfeeding and the Gendering of Infant Care." In *Beyond Health, Beyond Choice: Breastfeeding Constraints and Realities*, edited by Paige Hall Smith, Bernice L. Hausman, and Miram Labbok, 133–43. New Brunswick, NJ: Rutgers University Press.

– 2012b. "Is Breastfeeding Truly Cost Free? Income Consequences of Breastfeeding for Women." *American Sociological Review* 77, no. 2: 244–67.

Roberts, Dorothy. (1997) 2017. *Killing the Black Body: Race, Reproduction, and the Meaning of Liberty*. 2nd Vintage Books ed. New York: Vintage Books.

Robinson, Fiona. 2011. *The Ethics of Care: A Feminist Approach to Human Security*. Philadelphia: Temple University Press.

Robinson, Kathryn. 2009. *Gender, Islam and Democracy in Indonesia*. London: Routledge.

Rodgers, Kathleen. 2010. "'Anger Is Why We're All Here': Mobilizing and Managing Emotions in a Professional Activist Organization." *Social Movement Studies* 9, no. 3: 273–91. https://doi.org/10.1080/14742837.2010.493660.

Ron, Amos S., and Dallen Timothy. 2013. "The Land of Milk and Honey: Biblical Foods, Heritage and Holy Land Tourism." *Journal of Heritage Tourism* 8, nos. 2–3: 234–47. https://doi.org/10.1080/1743873X.2013.767817.

Rosin, Hanna. 2009. "The Case against Breast-Feeding." *Atlantic*, 1 April 2009. https://www.theatlantic.com/magazine/archive/2009/04/the-case-against-breast-feeding/307311.

Rousseau, Jean-Jacques. (1782) 2004. *The Confessions of Jean-Jacques Rousseau – Complete*. Project Gutenberg ebook. http://www.gutenberg.org/ebooks/3913.

– (1762) 2011. *Émile, or On Education*. Translated by Barbara Foxley. Project Gutenberg ebook. https://www.gutenberg.org/files/5427/5427-h/5427-h.htm.

Rushing, Sara. 2020. *The Virtues of Vulnerability: Humility, Autonomy, and Citizen-Subjectivity*. Oxford: Oxford University Press.

Salmon, Marylynn. 1994. "The Cultural Significance of Breastfeeding and Infant Care in Early Modern England and America." *Journal of Social History* 28, no. 2: 247–69. https://doi.org/10.1353/jsh/28.2.247.

Sandre-Pereira, Gilza. 2005. "La Leche League: Des Femmes Pour l'allaitement Maternel (1956–2004)." *CLIO: Histoire, Femmes et Sociétés* 21: 174–87.

Saurette, Paul, and Kelly Gordon. 2015. *The Changing Voice of the Anti-Abortion Movement: The Rise of "Pro-Woman" Rhetoric in Canada and the United States.* Toronto: University of Toronto Press.

Scariati, Paula D., Laurence M. Grummer-Strawn, and Sara Beck Fein. 1997. "A Longitudinal Analysis of Infant Morbidity and the Extent of Breastfeeding in the United States." *Pediatrics* 99, no. 6: article e5. https://doi.org/10.1542/peds.99.6.e5.

Schiebinger, Londa. 1993. "Why Mammals Are Called Mammals: Gender Politics in Eighteenth-Century Natural History." *American Historical Review* 98, no. 2: 382–411. https://doi.org/10.1086/ahr/98.2.382.

Scott, Joan Wallach. 1989. "French Feminists and the Rights of 'Man': Olympe de Gouges's Declarations." *History Workshop*, no. 28: 1–21.

Simons, Patricia. 2015. "The Crone, the Witch, and the Library: The Intersection of Classical Fantasy with Christian Vice during the Italian Renaissance." In *Receptions of Antiquity, Constructions of Gender in European Art, 1300–1600*, edited by Marice Rose and Alison C. Poe, 264–304. Leiden: Brill. https://doi.org/10.1163/9789004289697_010.

Singer, Merrill. 1995. "Beyond the Ivory Tower: Critical Praxis in Medical Anthropology." *Medical Anthropology Quarterly* 9, no. 1: 80–106.

Singla, Mani, Sushma Malik, Charusheela Sujit Korday, and Ashutosh Abhimanyu Paldiwal. 2018. "Weight Loss and/or Hypernatraemia in Inadequately Breastfed Term Neonates Having Non-Haemolytic Unconjugated Hyperbilirubinaemia." *Journal of Clinical & Diagnostic Research* 12, no. 1: 1–4. https://doi.org/10.7860/jcdr/2018/31791.11066.

Sinigaglia, Corrado, and Giacomo Rizzolatti. 2011. "Through the Looking Glass: Self and Others." *Consciousness and Cognition* 20: 64–74. https://doi.org/10.1016/j.concog.2010.11.012.

Smedley, Audrey, and Brian D. Smedley. 2005. "Race as Biology Is Fiction, Racism as a Social Problem Is Real: Anthropological and Historical Perspectives on the Social Construction of Race." *American Psychologist* 60, no. 1: 16–26.

Smith, Paige Hall. 2018. "Social Justice at the Core of Breastfeeding Protection, Promotion and Support: A Conceptualization." *Journal of Human Lactation* 34, no. 2: 220–5. https://doi.org/10.1177/0890334418758660.

Snow, David A., E. Burke Rochford, Steven K. Worden, and Robert D. Benford. 1986. "Frame Alignment Processes, Micromobilization, and Movement Participation." *American Sociological Review* 51, no. 4: 464–81.

Soldi, Antonella, Paola Tonetto, Alessia Varalda, and Enrico Bertino. 2011. "Neonatal Jaundice and Human Milk." *Journal of Maternal-Fetal & Neonatal Medicine* 24, no. S1: 85–7. https://doi.org/10.3109/14767058.2011.607612.

Sophia. 1739. *Woman not Inferior to Man: Or, a Short and Modest Vindication of the Natural Right of the Fair-Sex to a Perfect Equality of Power, Dignity and Esteem with the Men*. A Celebration of Women Writers website, edited by Mary Mark Ockerbloom. https://digital.library.upenn.edu/women/sophia/woman/woman.html.

– 1740. *Woman's Superior Excellence over Man: Or, a Reply to the Author of a Late Treatise, Entitled, Man Superior to Woman*. London: Printed for John Hawkins, at the Falcon in St Paul's Church-Yard. https://books.google.ca/books/edition/Woman_s_superior_excellence_over_Man_or/gbRgAAAAcAAJ.

Spain, Daphne. 2011. "Women's Rights and Gendered Spaces in 1970s Boston." *Frontiers: A Journal of Women Studies* 32, no. 1: 152–78. https://doi.org/10.5250/fronjwomestud.32.1.0152.

Spock, Benjamin. 1946. *The Common Sense Book of Baby and Child Care*. New York: Duell, Sloan and Pearce.

Stark, Rodney. 2001. "Reconceptualizing Religion, Magic, and Science." *Review of Religious Research* 43, no. 2: 101–20. https://doi.org/10.2307/3512057.

Steinbeck, John. 1939. *The Grapes of Wrath*. New York: Viking.

Stern, Philip D. 1992. "The Origin and Significance of 'The Land Flowing with Milk and Honey.'" *Vetus Testamentum* 42, no. 4: 554–7. https://doi.org/10.1163/15685330-042-04-09.

Stevens, Emily E., Thelma E. Patrick, and Rita Pickler. 2009. "A History of Infant Feeding." *Journal of Perinatal Education* 18, no. 2: 32–9. https://doi.org/10.1624/105812409X426314.

Stoller, Melissa Kaleta. 1995. "The Obstetric Pelvis and Mechanism of Labor in Nonhuman Primates." PhD diss., University of Chicago. ProQuest Dissertations. https://search.proquest.com/docview/304251435.

Stuebe, Alison. 2009. "The Risks of Not Breastfeeding for Mothers and Infants." *Reviews in Obstetrics and Gynecology* 2, no. 4: 222–31.

Sullivan, Margaret A. 2000. "The Witches of Dürer and Hans Baldung Grien," *Renaissance Quarterly* 53, no. 2: 333–401. https://doi.org/10.2307/2901872.

Sussman, George D. 1977. "The End of the Wet-Nursing Business in France, 1874–1914." *Journal of Family History* 2, no. 3: 237–58. https://doi.org/10.1177/036319907700200306.

Tapper, Josh. 2014. "Transgender Man Can Be Breastfeeding Coach." *Toronto Star*, 25 April 2014. https://www.thestar.com/life/health_wellness/2014/04/25/transgender_man_can_be_breastfeeding_coach.html.

Tarini, Beth A., Aaron E. Carroll, Colin M. Sox, and Dimitri A. Christakis. 2006. "Systematic Review of the Relationship between Early Introduction of Solid Foods to Infants and the Development of Allergic Disease." *Archives of Pediatrics & Adolescent Medicine* 160, no. 5: 502–7. https://doi.org/10.1001/archpedi.160.5.502.

Taylor, Erin N., and Lora Ebert Wallace. 2012. "For Shame: Feminism, Breast-feeding Advocacy, and Maternal Guilt." *Hypatia* 27, no. 1: 76–98. https://doi.org/10.1111/j.1527-2001.2011.01238.x.

Tessman, Lisa. 2010. "Idealizing Morality." *Hypatia* 25, no. 4: 797–824. https://doi.org/10.1111/j.1527-2001.2010.01125.x.

Thomas, William Isaac, and Dorothy Swaine Thomas. (1928) 1938. *The Child in America; Behavior Problems and Programs.* New York: A. A. Knopf.

Thulier, Diane. 2009. "Breastfeeding in America: A History of Influencing Factors." *Journal of Human Lactation* 25, no. 1: 85–94. https://doi.org/10.1177/0890334408324452.

Thulier, Diane, and Judith Mercer. 2009. "Variables Associated with Breastfeeding Duration." *Journal of Obstetric, Gynecologic & Neonatal Nursing* 38, no. 3: 259–68. https://doi.org/10.1111/j.1552-6909.2009.01021.x.

Tronto, Joan C. 1993. *Moral Boundaries: A Political Argument for an Ethic of Care.* New York: Routledge.

– 2009. "The 'Nanny' Question in Feminism." *Hypatia* 17, no. 2: 34–51.

– 2011. "A Feminist Democratic Ethics of Care and Global Care Workers: Citizenship and Responsibility." In *Feminist Ethics and Social Policy: Towards a New Global Political Economy of Care,* edited by Rianne Mahon and Fiona Robinson, 162–77. Vancouver: UBC Press.

– 2013. *Caring Democracy: Markets, Equality, and Justice.* New York: NYU Press.

Truth, Sojourner. 1851. "Ain't I a Woman?" *Anti-Slavery Bugle,* 21 June 1851.

Tuteur, Amy. 2019. "Formula Is Feminist" *Slate.* 20 March 2019. https://slate.com/technology/2019/03/bmj-decision-ban-formula-bad-for-women-not-based-on-evidence.html.

UN IGME (United Nations Inter-agency Group for Child Mortality Estimation). 2019. "CME Info - Child Mortality Estimates, United States, 1949–2018." https://childmortality.org/data/United%20States%20of%20America.

UNICEF. 2016. "Series from 'The Lancet' Provides More Evidence That Breast-feeding Is Lifesaving." Press release. 29 January 2016. https://www.unicef.org/media/media_89978.html.

UNICEF Innocenti Research Centre. 2005. *1990–2005: Celebrating the Innocenti Declaration on the Protection, Promotion and Support of Breastfeeding: Past Achievements, Present Challenges and the Way Forward for Infant and Young Child Feeding,* edited by Penny Van Esterik. Florence: UNICEF Innocenti Research Centre. https://www.unicef.org/nutrition/files/Innocenti_plus15_BreastfeedingReport.pdf.

US BLS (United States Bureau of Labor Statistics). 2020. "Labor Force Participation Rate – Women." LNS11300002. FRED (Federal Reserve Bank of St. Louis). Accessed 2 July 2020. https://fred.stlouisfed.org/series/lns11300002.

US Bureau of the Census. 1960. *Historical Statistics of the United States: Colonial Times to 1957*. A Statistical Abstract Supplement. Washington, DC.

USCS (US Cancer Statistics). 2020. "Leading Cancer Cases and Deaths, All Races/ Ethnicities, Male and Female, 2017." USCS Data Visualizations Tool. US Department of Health and Human Services, Centers for Disease Control and Prevention and National Cancer Institute, June 2020. https://gis.cdc.gov/Cancer/ USCS/DataViz.html.

Van Esterik, Penny. 1989. *Beyond the Breast-Bottle Controversy*. New Brunswick, NJ: Rutgers University Press.

Vltchek, Andre. 2012. *Indonesia: Archipelago of Fear*. London: Pluto Press. Kobo.

Waite, Linda J. 1976. "Working Wives: 1940–1960." *American Sociological Review* 41: 65–80.

Warner, Marina. 1985. *Alone of All Her Sex: The Myth and Cult of the Virgin Mary*. London: Picador.

Watson, Amanda D. 2020. *The Juggling Mother: Coming Undone in the Age of Anxiety*. Vancouver: UBC Press.

Watson, Amanda D., and Corinne L. Mason. 2015. "Power of the First Hour." *International Feminist Journal of Politics* 17, no. 4: 573–94. https://doi.org/10.1080/146 16742.2015.1080908.

Webb Girard, Aimee, Anne Cherobon, Samwel Mbugua, Elizabeth Kamau Mbuthia, Allison Amin, and Daniel W. Sellen. 2012. "Food Insecurity Is Associated with Attitudes towards Exclusive Breastfeeding among Women in Urban Kenya." *Maternal & Child Nutrition* 8, no. 2: 199–214. https://doi.org/10.1111/ j.1740-8709.2010.00272.x.

Weintraub, Karen. 2016. "20 Years after Dolly the Sheep Led the Way – Where Is Cloning Now?" *Scientific American*, 5 July 2016. https://www.scientificamerican. com/article/20-years-after-dolly-the-sheep-led-the-way-where-is-cloning-now.

Weiss, Penny A. 1987. "Rousseau, Antifeminism, and Woman's Nature." *Political Theory* 15, no. 1: 81–98. https://doi.org/10.1177/0090591787015001005.

Weiss, Penny, and Anne Harper. 1990. "Rousseau's Political Defense of the Sex-Roled Family." *Hypatia* 5, no. 3: 90–109. https://doi.org/10.1111/j.1527-2001.1990. tb00607.x.

Weiss, Sarah. 2017. "Rangda and the Goddess Durga in Bali." *Fieldwork in Religion* 12, no. 1: 50–77.

West, Emily, and R.J. Knight. 2017. "Mothers' Milk: Slavery, Wet-Nursing, and Black and White Women in the Antebellum South." *Journal of Southern History* 83, no. 1: 37–68. https://doi.org/10.1353/soh.2017.0001.

WHA (World Health Assembly). 1981. "Thirty-Fourth World Health Assembly, Geneva, 4–22 May 1981: Verbatim Records of Plenary Meetings, Reports of Committees." Document No. WHA34/1981/REC/2. World Health Organization, Geneva. https://apps.who.int/iris/handle/10665/155680.

White, Stephen K. 2017. *A Democratic Bearing: Admirable Citizens, Uneven Injustice, and Critical Theory*. Cambridge: Cambridge University Press.

WHO (World Health Organization). 2014. "Indonesia's Breastfeeding Challenge Is Echoed the World Over." *Bulletin of the World Health Organization*, April 2014.

– 2020. "Infant and Young Child Feeding." 24 August 2020. https://www.who.int/news-room/fact-sheets/detail/infant-and-young-child-feeding.

WHO and UNICEF. n.d. "Ten Steps to Successful Breastfeeding." Accessed 9 March 2021. https://www.who.int/activities/promoting-baby-friendly-hospitals/ten-steps-to-successful-breastfeeding.

Wickes, Ian G. 1953. "A History of Infant Feeding." *Archives of Disease in Childhood* 28, no. 138: 151–8.

"WIC Program Overview and History." 2018. National WIC Association. https://www.nwica.org/overview-and-history.

Wiessinger, Diane. 1996. "Watch Your Language!" *Journal of Human Lactation* 12, no. 1: 1–4. https://doi.org/10.1177/089033449601200102.

Wiessinger, Diane, Diana West, and Teresa Pitman. 2010. *The Womanly Art of Breastfeeding*. 8th ed. New York: Ballantine Books.

Williams, Cicely. (1939) 1986. "Milk and Murder." In *Milk and Murder*, 1–5. Penang, Malaysia: International Organization of Consumers Unions and International Baby Food Action Network.

Williams, Zoe. 2013. "Baby Health Crisis in Indonesia as Formula Companies Push Products." *Guardian*, 15 February 2013, World News. http://www.theguardian.com/world/2013/feb/15/babies-health-formula-indonesia-breastfeeding.

Wise, Cat. 2011. "New Indonesia Law: Allow Breastfeeding, or Face Punishment." *PBS NewsHour*, 5 July 2011, Health. https://www.pbs.org/newshour/health/in-indonesia-allow-breast-feeding-or-face-punishment.

Wolf, Jacqueline. 2001. *Don't Kill Your Baby: Public Health and the Decline of Breastfeeding in the Nineteenth and Twentieth Centuries*. Columbus: Ohio State University Press.

– 2003. "Low Breastfeeding Rates and Public Health in the United States." *American Journal of Public Health* 93, no. 12: 2000–10.

– 2006. "What Feminists Can Do for Breastfeeding and What Breastfeeding Can Do for Feminists." *Signs: Journal of Women in Culture and Society* 31, no. 2: 397–424.

Wolf, Joan B. 2007. "Is Breast Really Best? Risk and Total Motherhood in the National Breastfeeding Awareness Campaign." *Journal of Health Politics, Policy and Law* 32, no. 4: 595–636. https://doi.org/10.1215/03616878-2007-018.

– 2010. *Is Breast Best: Taking on the Breastfeeding Experts and the New High Stakes of Motherhood*. New York: NYU Press.

– 2013. "The Politics of Dissent." *Journal of Women, Politics & Policy* 34, no. 4: 306–16. https://doi.org/10.1080/1554477X.2013.835646.

– 2018. *Marketing of Breast-milk Substitutes: National Implementation of the International Code: Status Report*. Geneva: World Health Organization. https://www.who.int/nutrition/publications/infantfeeding/code_report2018.pdf.

Wright, Anne L., Catherine J. Holberg, Lynn M. Taussig, and Fernando D. Martinez. 1995. "Relationship of Infant Feeding to Recurrent Wheezing at Age 6 Years." *Archives of Pediatrics and Adolescent Medicine* 149, no. 7: 758–63. https://doi.org/10.1001/archpedi.1995.02170200048006.

Yi, Beh Lih. 2019. "Lack of Breastfeeding Costs Global Economy Nearly $1B Every Day." Global News, 12 July 2019. https://globalnews.ca/news/5489076/breastfeeding-global-economy-research.

Young, Iris Marion. 2005. *On Female Body Experience: "Throwing Like a Girl" and Other Essays*. New York: Oxford University Press. Kobo.

Zarshenas, Mahnaz, Yun Zhao, Colin W. Binns, and Jane A. Scott. 2018. "Baby-Friendly Hospital Practices Are Associated with Duration of Full Breastfeeding in Primiparous But Not Multiparous Iranian Women." *Maternal and Child Nutrition* 14, no. 3: e12583. https://doi.org/10.1111/mcn.12583.

Zika, Charles. 2007. *The Appearance of Witchcraft: Print and Visual Culture in Sixteenth-Century Europe*. New York: Routledge.

Index